Feeling F

CW00839175

Judy Chandler
and
Marguerite Childs

Adapted by
Sharon Goodyer

Longman

We are grateful to the following for permission
to reproduce photographs: National Dairy
Council, page 39; Optical Information Council,
page 16; Picturepoint, page 6 below; David
Richardson, page 71; Terry Williams, page 6
above.
Unless otherwise credited, all other photographs
are by Alan Trussell-Cullen.

We should like to acknowledge the help of
the Health Education Council and its
pamphlets in the preparation of this book.

LONGMAN GROUP LIMITED
Longman House, Burnt Mill, Harlow, Essex CM20 2JE, England
and Associated Companies throughout the World

This edition © Longman Group Limited 1985
All rights reserved. No part of this publication
may be reproduced, stored in a retrieval system,
or transmitted in any form or by any means, electronic,
mechanical, photocopying, recording or otherwise,
without the prior written permission of the Publishers.

First published by Longman Paul Ltd 1983
UK adapted edition first published 1985
ISBN 0 582 20633 2

Produced by Longman Group (FE) Ltd
Printed in Hong Kong

Illustrated by Cindy Hunnam

The authors have adapted in this book many
ideas, concepts, and topics for the teaching of
Health Education that they first developed and
trialled at the New Zealand Correspondence School.

Contents

Introduction

Do you want to **look good, feel fine,** and **enjoy life**? If you do, this book is for you. Like most people, you want to:
    be in charge of your own life
    have fun, and not be bored
    be attractive to your friends

have plenty of energy
enjoy your food
wake up feeling great
and be contented with yourself.
You will want these things now, and for the rest of your life. How can you manage this?

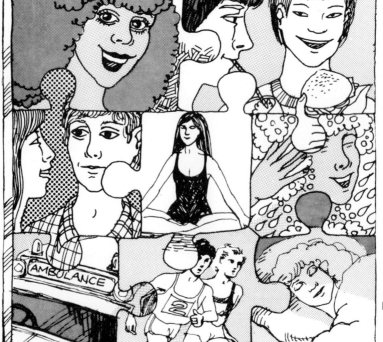

Being contented with yourself

Keeping moving

Knowing the dangers

Eating sensibly

Caring for your body— inside and out

Keeping in shape

Fit it all together

If all the pieces are in the picture it means you will find that life is a lot more fun. You will be healthy, and happier too. The pieces fit together if you:

- enjoy variety in your eating and are the right weight
- keep yourself clean—inside and outside
- enjoy exercise regularly
- get the right amount of sleep
- know how to cope with stress
- have a satisfying hobby
- don't smoke
- make an informed decision about drinking alcohol
- know how to keep yourself safe from disease.

You might need to make some changes in your lifestyle if you are to be healthy. This book will show you how to make these changes. But *you* have to decide. You are responsible for your own health choices. No one else can make you change.

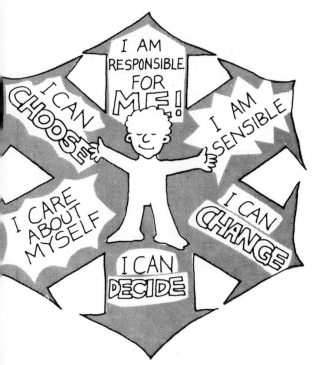

ACTIVITY

How healthy are you? Here is a health and lifestyle quiz to help you decide what to change! Write your answer alongside the number of each question in your exercise book.

In the past 24 hours have you:

1. Had at least two helpings of vegetables?
2. Walked fast for at least two km?
3. Eaten any sweets?
4. Smoked any cigarettes?
5. Showered, bathed, or washed all over?
6. Got a bit drunk?
7. Had at least half an hour's exercise?

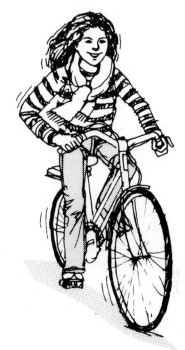

8. Had at least eight hours' sleep?
9. Had two or more helpings of fried food?
10. Spent a lot of time feeling upset or angry?
11. Had a filling breakfast including cereal or bread (or toast)?
12. Relaxed with your family or friends?
13. Worked on a hobby?
14. Eaten cake or sweet biscuits for snacks?
15. Taken vitamin tablets?
16. Had a soft drink to drink?
17. Taken pills or medicine not prescribed by the doctor?
18. Cleaned your teeth at least twice?
19. Sprinkled salt on your food?
20. Washed your hands before eating?

In your spare time do you (answer 'usually', 'rarely', or 'never'):

21 Watch TV?
22 Work on a hobby?
23 Call up or visit friends?
24 Get some exercise?
25 Do as little as possible?

When you're with your family or friends do you (usually, rarely, or never):

26 Have a fight or an argument?
27 Do something else energetic (dancing, skating, walking, swimming, hiking)?
28 Get a bit drunk?
29 Just sit around?
30 Eat a lot?

Now check your answers:

If you wrote **No** for any of these numbers: 1, 2, 5, 7, 8, 11, 12, 13, 18, and 20 . . .

If you wrote **Yes** for any of these numbers: 3, 4, 6, 9, 10, 14, 15, 16, 17, and 19 . . .

If you wrote **Usually** for any of these numbers: 21, 25, 26, 28, 29, and 30 . . .

If you wrote **Rarely** for any of these numbers: 22, 23, 24, and 27 . . .

. . . you can decide to make changes for a healthier and happier you.

In your exercise book underline the choices you gave which are *good* for your health. In the rest of this book you will find out more about the good health choices you can make.

Look back at your list. Decide on *one* change you can make today. (You can make other changes later.) Make a **Contract** with yourself. It could be like the one on the right.

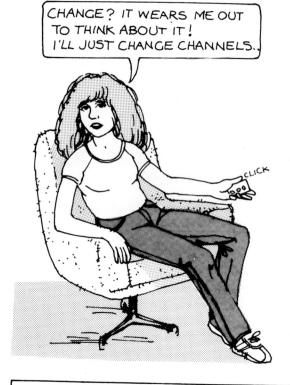

CHANGE? IT WEARS ME OUT TO THINK ABOUT IT! I'LL JUST CHANGE CHANNELS.

CLICK

CONTRACT
I Plan To:

Things I might do or excuses I might invent to stop me from doing this:

1
Clean scene

Looking good, feeling good, and enjoying life all start with looking after your body's container.

Riddle: What part of your body never stops growing, but never gets too big for you?
Clue: It is a magic coating!
Clue: It helps to make you waterproof.
Clue: It helps to control your body's temperature and protects you from infection.
Clue: It helps to make you sensitive to touch, heat, cold, and pain.
Clue: It is a most important ingredient in attracting others to you.

There is only one answer to this riddle. Of course you have guessed—it is your *skin*. Your skin is the magic coating which grows with you and stops the inside of your body from drying out.

Without waterproof skin you would be like a raisin! Skin also stops you absorbing extra water. Imagine if you got waterlogged everytime you had a bath or went for a swim.

Unbroken skin keeps bacteria out and protects you from infection.

Temperature control? Your skin cools you down by sweating and the blood vessels of your skin bring extra blood near the surface for cooling. (What colour does your face go when you get very hot?) Your skin helps to keep you warm too. When you get too cold the hairs on your skin stand up, trying to trap extra air to insulate you. The surface blood vessels close off, keeping the blood deep down inside where it is warm.

Nerves in your skin tell you what you are touching. Is it hot? Cold? Painful?

Skin also grows hair—on body and head—as well as toes and fingernails. When you see someone, you usually see their hair and their face first.

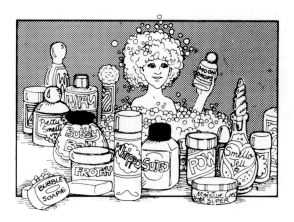

It makes sense to save your skin.

How do you look after your skin to keep it healthy and attractive? You look after it from the inside as well as from the outside. Looking after your skin like this is easy. It just becomes part of your everyday life.

FROM THE INSIDE

Sensible eating and drinking

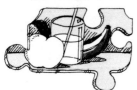

Eat a wide variety of food—plenty of raw fruit, vegetables, and cereals. Enjoy drinking water and fruit juices

Enough sleep

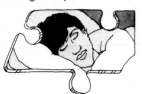

Tired people look tired, and their skin is dull and tired-looking too

No smoking

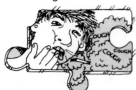

Smoking gives you bad breath and smelly clothes and stops you looking clean and fresh

Regular exercise

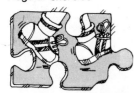

Exercise keeps the skin firm and elastic. Sweat unblocks pores and helps prevent spots

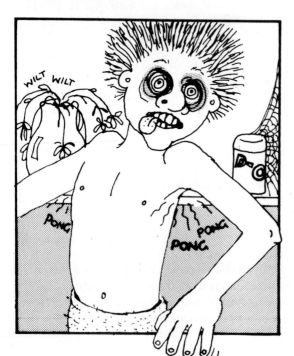

FROM THE OUTSIDE

Shower, bath, or wash all over every day

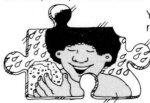

You need water and soap regularly, to remove:
stale sweat
dirt and grime
body grease
dead skin cells
bacteria
body odours

Protect your skin from the sun

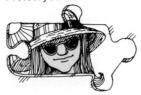

Sunshine can give you a healthy looking tan but sunburn ages and wrinkles skin

Other protection

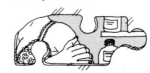

Skin may sometimes need moisturisers, creams, or ointments so it can feel and look good

Questions about skin

Q: I know that I need a deodorant. I don't want to stink of sweat. But I don't want to stink of scent either. Dad reckons that stick deodorants aren't strong enough for me. What can I do?

David

A: Try an anti-perspirant. Deodorants stop sweat smelling for some hours, while anti-perspirants partially stop the sweat glands secreting sweat. They are not able to stop the sweat completely.

Always put on a deodorant or an anti-perspirant when you have cooled down after your bath or shower. Don't expect to cover up stale sweat.

There are plenty of different brands, some with no perfume.

If any brand irritates your skin, give it up immediately. There are one or two allergy tested brands on the market. Read

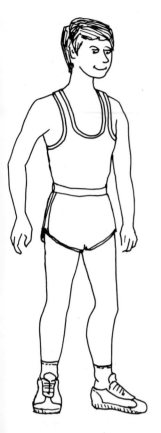

Hair: wash once a week at least. There are medicated shampoos for dandruff
Nose: 'fingering' spreads germs. Use a clean handkerchief or tissues
Teeth: clean morning and night, or better still after every meal

Armpits: wash every day

Crutch: wash every day

Hands: should always be washed both after going to the lavatory and before preparing food

Feet: wash daily. Cut toenails straight across, change socks or tights daily

Personal cleanliness will help you to avoid skin troubles and keep you smelling sweet

the label on deodorants and anti-perspirants carefully.

Q: Another question about smells! How often should I wash my clothes?

Kim

A: Change the clothes you wear next to your skin every single day. Wash clothes before they look dirty—if you're not sure, it's time to wash them. Follow the care-label instructions when washing. Outer clothes may need dry cleaning. They get smelly too.
   Remember that we wash clothes to get rid of smells, grease and grime, dead skin, and bacteria—in fact all the things that make your skin dirty. Your clothes are like your second skin. Dry them in the fresh air whenever you can. Sunlight kills germs too. It is a good idea to put your outer clothes in the fresh air to air them—often.

Q: Do I need cosmetics and lotions and things? They are very expensive but I do want to look as good as I can.

Sandy

A: Soap and water is still the best cosmetic. If your skin is dry and flaky, a moisturiser may help. Consumer tests have shown that the cheaper ones are just as good as the most expensive. Try the cheapest ones—the sort you buy at the supermarket or chain store—first.

Q: What causes acne? Why do teenagers get acne?

Just Interested

A: To understand the causes of acne you need to know a bit about the structure of the skin. The skin has two layers. The epidermis is the layer you can see. The dermis is the

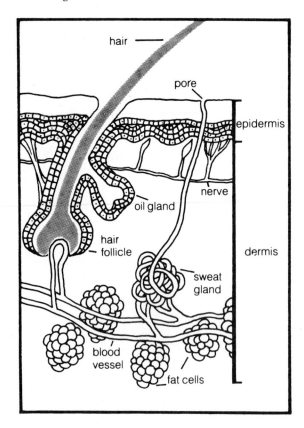

The structure of skin

The result is a tiny cyst or bump just below the skin surface. The plug may stretch the pore open and rise slightly above the skin surface. This is a blackhead. If the plug bursts the follicle, the dead cells and bacteria get into the deeper layers of skin and form a pimple or inflamed spot.

Doctors can help with special acne treatments. Let your doctor know that you want help now—not to wait until you 'grow out of it'.

The treatment can take time to work. Don't give up before it has had time to help you.

---

layer underneath. Inside the dermis are oil glands which put a thin coat of oil on each hair. Dead cells on the skin surface are shed all the time and replaced by new ones. The cells lining the hair follicles are also shed.

Many people believe that acne is caused by dirt, but neither dirt nor poor hygiene causes acne. Even blackheads get their colour from skin pigment, not dirt.* Acne starts below the skin. At puberty when there are lots of body changes going on, often the oil glands begin to work overtime. Also something goes wrong with the normal cell-shedding process. The cells are shed in greater numbers and they begin to stick together. These dead cells combine with oil and bacteria in the hair follicles, form a plug, and block the follicles up.

Q: How can I get rid of acne and pimples?
Fed-up

A: You're probably fed up with this answer too, but you *will* grow out of acne. (How often do you see an adult with acne?) That's not much comfort right now, so here's what you can do meanwhile:

- keep skin clean—wash gently with soap. Don't scrub and rub or you may do more damage
- get plenty of exercise—sweating helps unblock pores
- don't pick spots—you can spread infection and cause scarring
- eat plenty of fresh fruit and vegetables—some people find chocolate and fried foods make their acne worse
- avoid thick greasy creams and make-up, which can clog pores
- get rid of dandruff—it can make acne worse.

Chemists' lotions sometimes work but it is best to get your doctor to prescribe a lotion.

Because of body changes teenage girls may find that their skin is worse just before a period is due.

---

* Did you know albinos have no skin pigment? Is that why they don't get blackheads?

Hair care

Wash your hair at least once a week—to get rid of dead skin, as well as dirt, dust, and grease. Always use two lots of shampoo when you wash. Rinse thoroughly. Shampoo is easier to rinse out than soap.

Brush hair regularly. Brushing helps make hair shine. Even oily hair needs some brushing.

Wash your brush and comb every time you wash your hair.

If the ends of your hair are split, the only thing you can do is cut off the split ends.

Rinse hair after swimming to remove chlorine or salt.

Keep your hair trimmed—in a style that suits you. Ask your hairdresser for help and advice.

Questions about hair

Q: Greasy hair is my problem! Can you please tell me how to deal with it? Mum says I'll grow out of it but I need help *now!*

Sally

A: Greasy hair is a common problem. Most people do grow out of it, but remember that when you are a teenager your body is changing. That also means changes in hormones, the chemical messengers in your body. The new message is: produce more oil! So the glands *do* produce more oil and one of the places you notice it most is on your scalp and in your hair. All you can do is shampoo as often as your hair gets greasy. For some people this will be every day. Choose a shampoo for oily hair (though no one shampoo will decrease the rate of oil flow).

Q: Does home bleaching and tinting damage my hair?

Paula

A: Yes, it does. It is better to have it done professionally.

Q: What do I do about dandruff?

Susan

A: A small amount of flaking is normal. Everyone has to shed skin cells from their scalp. Use a conditioner for your hair type if it is dry.

For mild dandruff use a medicated shampoo. If it is very bad, buy special lotion from the chemist. Wash your brush and comb frequently. Don't borrow or lend brushes or combs—that's a good rule for everyone.

CASE STUDIES

Some skin stories

Darren tattooed LOVE on one hand and another design on his leg. Almost straight away he wished he hadn't. He tried rubbing salt into the skin until it bled. It was very painful. Then ulcers formed on his leg and stayed for three months. The tattoos were still just as obvious. In the end Darren had to have the tattoos removed by surgery. It cost several hundred pounds to have the operation done in a private hospital. National Health Service hospitals are too busy to take non-urgent cases.

Ann nearly stopped running because her skin got so sore and chafed. Her gym teacher said, 'Put Vaseline where your clothes rub. Always wear clean clothes, because stale perspiration can cause chafing too.' Ann found this advice worked. She also switched to cotton towelling shorts and top as she found cotton absorbed the perspiration better.

David used to get dreadful chilblains in the winter. His toes burnt and itched. He was very miserable. Then the doctor told him to keep warm and dry and do more exercise to improve his circulation. He had to wear shoes with enough room to move his toes. David found that it helped to warm up in a shower and then walk to school. David hardly noticed his chilblains all last winter.

Skin and sun

Our skin colour depends on the amount of pigment (called melanin) in the skin. Black people have more melanin in their skin than light-skinned people.

Everyone's skin has melanin-producing cells. When you stay out in the sun, melanin is produced to protect you from the burning rays of the sun (these burning rays are ultra-violet rays). A 'tan' is the result of the melanin production.

Some skin makes a lot of melanin. Other skin doesn't make very much. The skin of boy number 3 produces little melanin, so he needs to be careful in the sun. Otherwise, he burns

People who freckle easily need to stay out of the sun to avoid burning.

Freckles will fade gradually. It is unwise to try to bleach freckles. There is really no way to remove them safely. Freckles give a person's face 'character'.

There were only 1299 hours of bright sunshine in Birmingham in 1983. It is important that you go outside in what sunshine there is because the sun's ultra violet rays will help your skin make vitamin D. Your body will use this vitamin D to build and maintain strong bones and teeth.

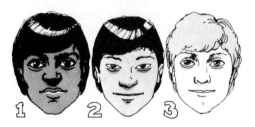

The skins of these boys have different amounts of melanin-producing cells

You don't have to live in the country to enjoy the sunshine!

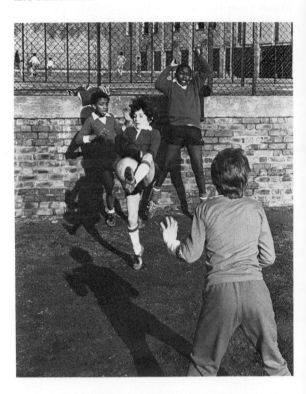

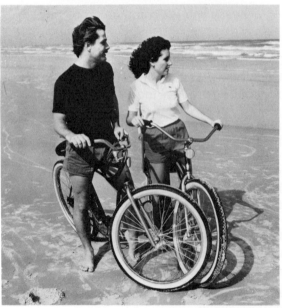

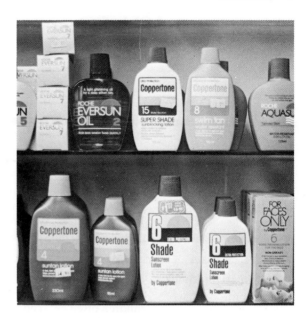

FIRST AID FOR SUNBURN

The best treatment for sunburn is probably a cool bath or shower. Some lotions will ease the pain. Ask your chemist.

Skin-saving tips

- Cover up when out for a long time in bright sunshine.
- Wear a hat, use a sunscreen. Some sunscreens have 'SPF' numbers. 'SPF' means Sun Protection Factor. The higher the number, the more ultra-violet rays will be screened out, and you can stay in the sun a little longer. Ask your chemist. People with fair skin always need to take special care, even with a sunscreen.
- Don't go to sleep in the sun.
- You can get extra-burnt when the sun is reflected off water or snow.
- You can still get burnt when you are busy doing something like sailing or gardening.
- You don't have to be hot to get burnt. You can get very burnt high up a snowy mountain.

Sunburn—it will make you look older!

The first result of too much sun is painful sunburn. Another result is skin that grows old before you do. Too much sun gives you wrinkles and tough leathery skin.

Too much sunshine can be harmful. In Kenya there are on average 2832 hours of bright sunshine each year. People in hot, sunny countries have dark skins which protect them from damage. But dark skinned people in Britain will not absorb enough sunlight to make all the vitamin D they need. So they must get more of their vitamin D from foods such as eggs, margarine, dairy foods and tinned fish.

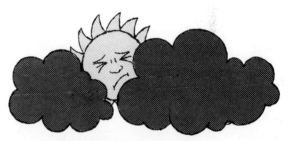

Are you getting enough vitamin D?

Do you spend most of the daylight hours indoors?

Do you cover most of your skin with clothes when you go out?

Do you eat any of the foods listed on the left?

Skinvaders and Skinfecters

Other things can damage skin:

Agent	Signs and symptoms	Treatment
Allergies ● eczema ● hives ● dermatitis	The skin reacts to certain substances by itching and developing a rash	Don't scratch! See chemist or doctor for 'anti-itch' treatment
Bacteria (germs) ● boils ● acne ● infected wounds	Bacteria multiply only when they can get in through a break in the skin. There is redness, swelling, and even pus. Bacterial infection is easily spread	A small skin infection can be treated with antiseptic. Infected wounds or bad acne or more than one boil may need treating with medication from the doctor
Fungi (fungal infection) ● ringworm ● athlete's foot	There are no 'worms' in ringworm. The fungus grows in a circle or ring. Young children often get scalp ringworm from the family cat. More on athlete's foot in Chapter 2	It is important to get a special lotion from the chemist or doctor. Never use home remedies
Insects ● lice (nits) ● fleas	These parasites can live off human blood! They cause itching of head or body, soreness, and their bites often get infected. Nits are the eggs of lice	Treatment includes precautions to stop the spread. Special lotions are needed

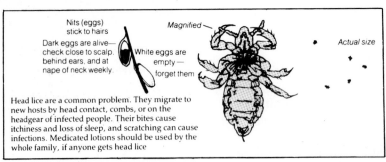

Nits (eggs) stick to hairs

Dark eggs are alive— check close to scalp, behind ears, and at nape of neck weekly.

White eggs are empty — forget them

Magnified

Actual size

Head lice are a common problem. They migrate to new hosts by head contact, combs, or on the headgear of infected people. Their bites cause itchiness and loss of sleep, and scratching can cause infections. Medicated lotions should be used by the whole family, if anyone gets head lice

Agent	Signs and symptoms	Treatment
Mites ● Scabies	Extreme itchiness. Female mite burrows into skin. The burrows may be seen as dark lines, especially in body folds and creases	Use medication as directed. Wash body surfaces of patient and contacts carefully. Disinfect underclothes and bedding, as scabies can spread easily

Agent	Signs and symptoms	Treatment
Viruses ● cold sores (herpes)	Blisters form on skin around mouth. They can also form on male and female genitals. Genital herpes is spread by sexual intercourse	Special lotion or cream from chemist. Seek medical help for genital herpes. There is no known cure—yet
● warts	Warts—growths—usually on hands	Some disappear by themselves, others can be removed by a doctor
● veruccae (plantar warts)	Veruccae are painful ingrowths on feet—sometimes hands	See doctor or clinic for treatment for veruccae—warts and veruccae can be treated in several different ways

ACTIVITIES

Discuss

1 Are first impressions important? Is it right to judge people by their outside appearance?

2 We cannot rely on a large number of hours of bright sunshine in this country. Why is it good to get outside and make the most of the sunshine we do get?

3 Suggest several activities which would get you outside on a chilly but sunny winter's day.

4 It is difficult to find a photo of someone with acne. Why is this? Can you find any?

5 Collect advertisements from papers and magazines for hair and skin care products. What do the advertisers suggest will happen to you if you use their products? What do you think the products *really* do?

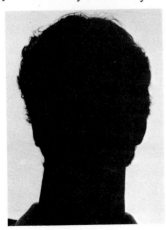

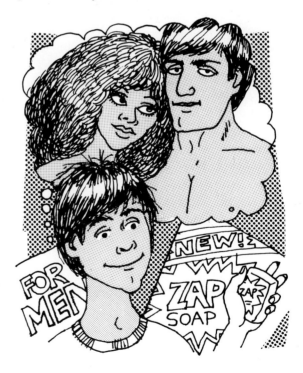

6   Make up a wordsearch. Fit as many of the important words from this chapter as you can across, down, or diagonally. See how many words your partner can find.

7   Ask your local Health Visitor to talk about skin infections in the community. Prepare questions to ask her or him.

8   Help others to learn about skin infections. Choose one topic from the chart on pages 8 and 9. Find out more about it! Ask teachers, at the library, at your local Health Education Service. Now make a pamphlet about your topic. It must have a clear message, be easy to read and understand, and eye-catching.

For You to Do

1   Chart your colouring. In your exercise book describe your hair, eye, and skin colouring and say how sensitive you are to the ultra-violet (burning) rays of the sun.

2   Find out which brands of sunscreens carry SPF (Sun Protection Factor) numbers. What are the numbers? Which would be best for you?

3   Design a hair shampoo user test to see which shampoo is best for greasy hair. Put the shampoos in plain bottles, coded, so your users won't be influenced by:
- the packaging
- brand names
- marketing gimmicks
- advertising claims
- personal preferences.

You will need to devise a score sheet. Users must use each shampoo at least three times. *Which?* magazine April 1983 will help you.

4   Here are the answers to a 'Clean Scene' quiz. You make up the questions! All the questions should be to do with you and your skin, of course.

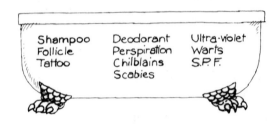

Shampoo	Deodorant	Ultra-violet
Follicle	Perspiration	Warts
Tattoo	Chilblains	S.P.F.
	Scabies	

The 'Clean Scene' answers. Make up a quiz with them

2
Top to toe

Listen carefully!

Guess what
- is more complicated than a stereo
- can tell the difference between treble and bass
- is a most delicate instrument
- contains a hammer and a drum
- is connected to the back of your nose and throat
- always comes in pairs
- has direct contact with your brain
- gets damaged by loud noise
- can be wiggled (by some people)
- is inside and outside your body
- keeps you balanced
- is sometimes seen wearing jewellery
- is a machine for picking up sound?

There is only one answer . . . your EARS!

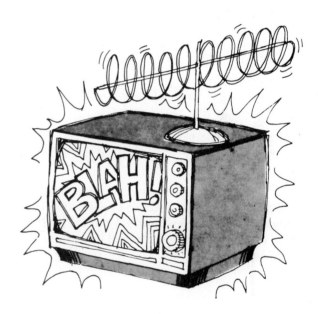

Noise

Noise is unwanted sound. It won't kill you—it can only drive you nuts or make you deaf. How can noise make you deaf? The energy in sound waves can cause damage to the eardrum, if it strikes hard enough or long enough. Noises can damage the nerves which carry sound messages to the brain, too.

Now hear this!

Hear the bad news about noise and hearing.

Fact   Teenagers often listen to high-powered stereo and electronic equipment. They live in a noisier world than their parents did. Many teenagers suffer hearing loss.

Fact   Everyone over 40 has some hearing loss.

Fact   Deafness comes on faster in people who have been exposed to large amounts of noise.

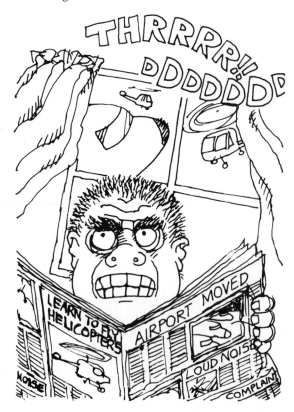

Fact   Very loud noise for even a short time will affect your ears. You can't hear properly. This wears off in a few hours, *but* if the high level of noise continues you will lose your hearing—permanently. You will become deaf.

Fact   Hearing loss is generally gradual.

Fact   Doctors cannot cure deafness caused by exposure to high levels of sound. As you probably know the strength or **intensity** of a sound is measured in **decibels** (dB). Silence is measured at 0 decibels.

We can't wipe out the sounds of jet planes, motor mowers, chain saws, or heavy trucks. But we can take some steps to protect our hearing.

- Turn down before tuning in! Listen to music at a lower volume. Be especially careful if you use earphones.
- Replace silencers on cars and motorbikes.
- Put a pad of plastic or rubber foam under noisy equipment—like a typewriter or cakemixer.

- Don't confuse your ears with too many sounds. Turn the radio off if no one is listening. Shut the door to keep out unwanted sounds. Remember continuous low level noise is as harmful as shorter, louder noise.
- Sit or stand further back at concerts. Put distance between you and the loudspeakers.
- Wear earmuffs if you have to work or play near loud noise. Employers are responsible for providing earmuffs for noisy jobs. *You* are responsible for wearing them.

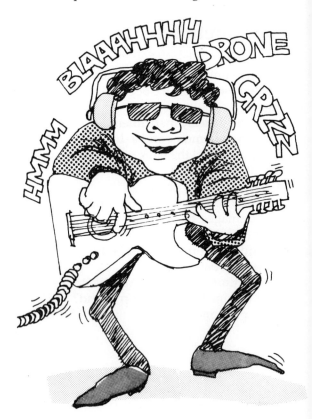

Looking after your ears

When you blow your nose, blow gently. Keep both nostrils open as you blow. Hold the bony part at the top of your nose. If you blow too hard, you may force bacteria-filled mucus up your eustachian tubes. This can give you earache.

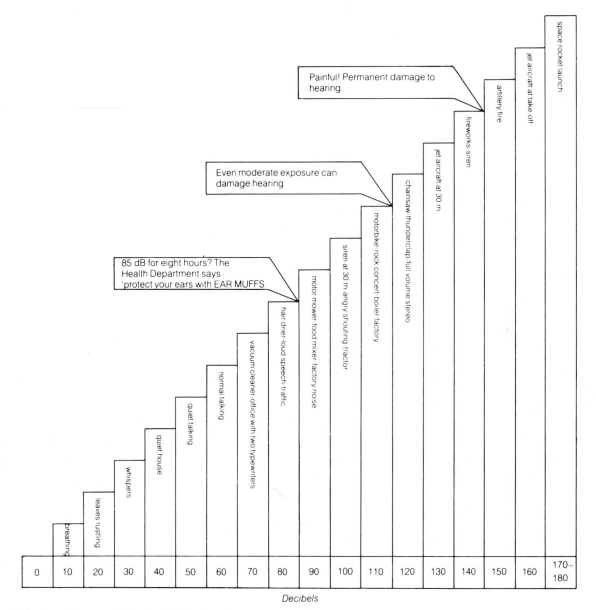

Painful! Permanent damage to hearing.

Even moderate exposure can damage hearing

85 dB for eight hours? The Health Department says 'protect your ears with EAR MUFFS.

space rocket launch

jet aircraft at take off

artillery fire

fireworks·siren

jet aircraft at 30 m

chainsaw·thunderclap·full volume stereo

motorbike·rock concert·boiler factory

siren at 30 m·angry shouting·tractor

motor mower·food mixer·factory noise

hair drier·loud speech·traffic

vacuum cleaner·office with two typewriters

normal talking

quiet talking

quiet house

whispers

leaves rustling

breathing

| 0 | 10 | 20 | 30 | 40 | 50 | 60 | 70 | 80 | 90 | 100 | 110 | 120 | 130 | 140 | 150 | 160 | 170–180 |

Decibels

This chart shows you the decibel levels of common sounds

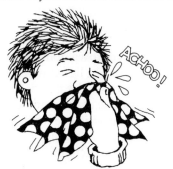

Clean in and around your ears every day using a warm, soapy flannel. Don't put things like pencils, cottonbuds, or hairclips into your ears—you could damage your eardrum. Hitting someone on the ear can damage the eardrum too.

If you can't hear well, or get noises in your ears, see your doctor. Often all that is wrong is a build-up of wax in your ears. This is easy to syringe out.

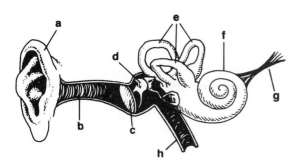

a external ear—collects sound waves

b wax and hairs—trap dirt or insects that might harm the middle or inner ear

c ear drum—sound waves make it vibrate

d three small bones in a row (the arrow points to the first)—magnify the vibrations

e three semicircular canals—turning your head makes the liquid in these canals move. Sensory cells in the canal walls send messages to your brain. This is how we keep our balance, and why ear problems can make us feel giddy

f liquid-filled 'snail'—the little bone like a stirrup vibrates against this, the liquid moves back and forth and sensory cells send sound messages to the brain

g the auditory nerve—sound and balance messages pass along here

h eustachian tube—goes from middle ear to the throat. If air pressure builds up on one side of the eardrum (skin diving, in a plane) it might burst. Make the pressure equal by opening your mouth and swallowing.

How an ear works—inside and out

Don't try to pierce your ears yourself. And don't let your friends do it for you. Go to a specialist. If you do get your ears pierced be very careful about keeping the area clean. Don't touch with dirty hands or you might get your ears infected.

Protect your ears from noise.

Watch out—eyes at risk!

What can damage your eyes? Which of these are dangerous?

1 rubbing your eyes
2 knitting needles and sharp scissors
3 fireworks
4 splashing liquids such as household bleaches and cleaners
5 flying chips from a chainsaw
6 ski-ing or walking in the snow without goggles or dark glasses
7 eye make-up
8 wind-blown dust and dirt
9 looking at the sun
10 air guns, darts, bows and arrows
11 crying
12 TV
13 contact lenses
14 looking at bright lights such as welding

All of these can damage your eyes, *except:*

1 Unless you rub your eyes a lot. This may be a sign that you need glasses
7 Unless you are allergic to it. Eye make-up must be removed at bed-time
11 Crying just makes your eyes *look* awful
12 Sensible TV viewing isn't harmful
13 Properly fitted and looked-after contact lenses are safe.

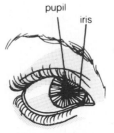 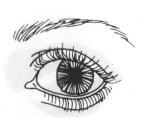

The pupil is a hole at the centre of the iris

Your eyes have built-in protection. (What do eyelids and eyebrows do for you?) There is protection from bright lights too. Light gets into your eye through the pupil. (What colour are pupils?) The size of the pupil controls how much light gets into the eye. (What size are pupils in bright light? Dim light?) Tears are a slightly salty fluid which has some

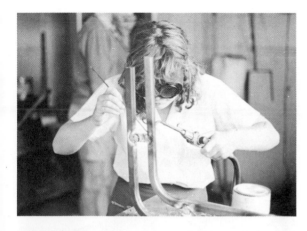

'At our school we wear safety goggles in the workshop when we use the machines. We try to prevent accidents to eyes. You can protect your eyes too, by wearing snow goggles in the snow, and never looking at the sun—even when you're wearing sun glasses. Direct sun can destroy some cells in your retina. Reading a book in strong sun isn't a good idea either. Save your sight!

'You have only one pair of eyes. You can't get another pair. When you watch TV make sure there's a light on in the room, otherwise there's too much contrast. Focus the picture clearly. Don't sit too close and rest your eyes now and then. Experts agree that watching TV isn't harmful as long as you are sensible.

'Eyestrain happens when your eyes are tired from
- not using them properly
- vision defects
- eye disorders.

You will know you have eyestrain if you have:
- aching or pains in the eyes
- a hot, scratchy feeling in your eyelids
- blurred vision, dizziness
- headaches a lot.

Get help!'

Who needs help for eye care?

Of course if you have an accident to your eyes you will get medical help straight away from your own doctor or the Accident and Emergency Department at the nearest hospital.

Anyone else who
- has difficulty focusing on near or far-away objects
- rubs eyes a lot
- gets sore eyes or has red-looking eyes or eyelids
- stumbles over small objects
- has headaches often
- is very sensitive to light
- has blurred vision
- screws up eyes when trying to see something
- is diabetic

may need an eye test.

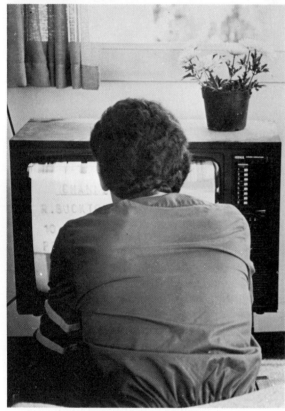

germ-killing powers. (If you get something in your eye, why does it water? How does this help?)

Some students made a study of eyes and eye care. Here are some of the things they found out.

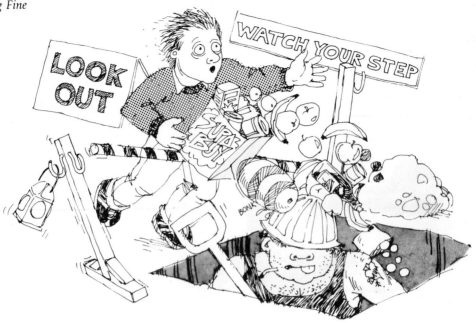

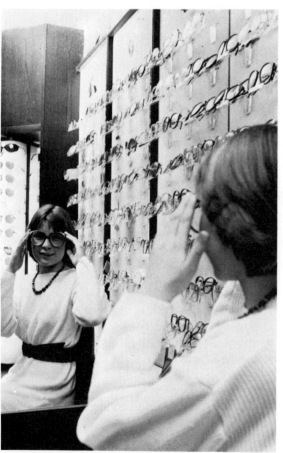

Who to see

There are several different sorts of eye-care professionals.

The first person you see is often your usual doctor. Your doctor may treat you for certain eye conditions, but could refer you to an eye specialist (ophthalmologist).

Ophthalmologist

An ophthalmologist (say off-thal-mollo-jist) is a doctor who specialises in eye diseases and does eye operations.

Ophthalmologists also test eyes and write prescriptions for glasses and contact lenses. You must be referred to these specialist doctors by your own doctor.

Opticians

Opticians are trained to examine and test your eyes as well as to make and fit glasses from a prescription.

You will find doctor's names in the Yellow Pages phone directory under 'Physicians and surgeons'. Or you can get a list of family doctors from main libraries and post offices. You can find the names of opticians in the Yellow Pages too.

Eye Care (I Care)

Something in your eye? Here is what to do.

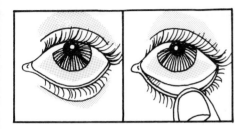

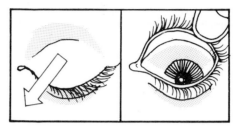

Foreign Bodies

To remove a bit of dust or grit from the eye, part the eyelids carefully and lift the particle off gently with the clean corner of a handkerchief or paper tissue. It is often best to get someone else to remove foreign bodies.

Do not attempt to remove the grit
● If it is over the pupil.
● If it does not lift off easily.
● If there is blood anywhere in the eye.
In these cases see your doctor as soon as possible.

Foreign body under upper eyelid: Holding eyelashes, draw upper lid gently over lower lid. This makes the eye water, which may wash out the grit. If this does not work, ask the person to look down. Then, still holding the lashes, gently roll the eyelid up and lift the grit off with the clean corner of a handkerchief or paper tissue.

Foreign body under lower eyelid: With the person looking up, gently pull eyelid out and down. Lift off the grit.

Chemical Injuries

Splashes of a chemical (either acid or alkali) in the eye cause burns which can be very serious.

Immediate first aid is vital. The eye must be washed with a gentle continuous stream of water for at least five minutes. Pour water from a jug or tea pot (an eye glass is not big enough) holding it a few centimetres away from the eye. You may need help to keep the eye open so that the water runs over the whole eyeball.

See your doctor immediately afterwards.

From a New Zealand Department of Health pamphlet, Mind Your Eye

Injury to eyes

If eyes are accidentally bruised by a ball or a fist, there can be inside damage. See your doctor to check that there is no damage. Always see your doctor if your eye is injured by a sharp object. It can be serious.

Eye infections

If your eyes are swollen, red, discharging pus, or painful, see your doctor. Some eye infections are very contagious (catching).

Eye diseases

Two common eye diseases are:

Styes   A stye is a tiny abscess in the base of an eyelash.

Conjunctivitis   The membrane lining the eyelids gets inflamed. The eye becomes red and feels gritty. Eyelids are often stuck together in the morning.

Eye wear

Contact lenses

Contact lenses take extra care. How do you choose between soft and hard lenses? Consult your eye-care specialist. Some eye vision problems can be corrected only with hard contact lenses. If you have a choice, keep these tips in mind: Hard lenses take more time to get used to, but provide sharper vision than soft lenses. Hard lenses can last forever if they're properly cared for. Soft lenses are comfortable, but they must be replaced as often as every one or two years.

Hard lenses must be cleaned and disinfected daily with a special solution. Soft lenses require more attention.

Contacts have some advantages over glasses. They give you more side vision, they don't steam up or streak in rain. And they don't usually fall off during strenuous activity. Of course contact lenses are more expensive, and they do get lost *sometimes*. You can insure contact lenses against loss.

Glasses

Choose a frame that feels smooth and sturdy—be sure to check out the hinges. Metal frames need an overall even lustre and smoothly finished joints. Plastic frames need a hard, glossy finish without 'bubbles'. Look for hinges that are recessed into the frame with the edges polished smooth.

Try on frames for fit. They're too snug if they press tightly against your nose, cheeks, temples or over your ears. And if the glasses slip off when you lean over, they're obviously too loose. In either case, ask for an adjustment.

Plastic lenses are lighter than glass but require extra care because they scratch more easily. Always wash lenses clean with soap and warm water.

If your prescription is very strong, choose glass lenses; they'll look less thick. Looking-good advice: match the colour of the frame to your complexion.

Big glasses must have plastic lenses. Glass lenses would be too heavy. Glass lenses can be **photochromic**, that is, they darken in bright light.

Hardened glass can be used in prescription glasses. This is a special glass which will not shatter and is a safety measure for people who have an active life.

Save your smile

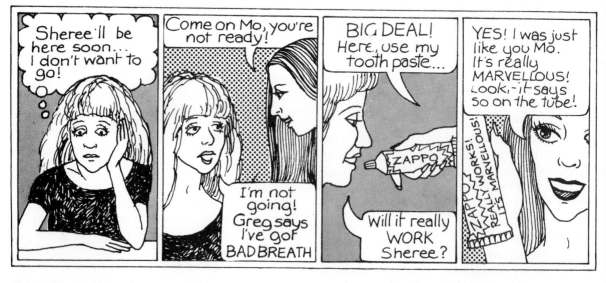

Does Sharon's toothpaste work?
Does Jo begin to smile?
Do boys get bad breath?
Do teenagers like smiles?
How can you look after teeth *and* have fresh breath?

You'll find the answers on the next few pages.

Save your smile by caring for your teeth and gums. Plaque is the enemy. Plaque is a thin sticky film that makes your teeth feel dirty and furry when they haven't been brushed. If you don't get rid of plaque every day, you will get dental decay (caries), bleeding gums, and even bad breath. (Another name for bad breath is halitosis.

There are other causes of bad breath. Infections of the throat and digestive tract, smoking, and some foods can make your breath smell.) Eventually your teeth may loosen in your gums—all because of plaque.

Plaque is made up of bacteria. Within minutes of your eating sugar, these bacteria produce an acid which attacks your teeth and gums. There are FOUR things you can do to prevent this:

- get rid of plaque
- watch your diet
- toughen your teeth
- visit your dentist.

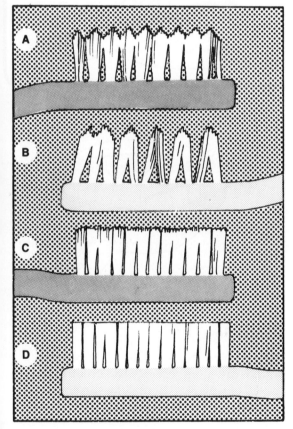

Just as trim *style* is important, so is trim *quality*. For example: **A** Tufted and serrated: ragged; **B** Angle-tufted: ragged; **C** Straight, ragged; **D** Straight: good

from Consumer *198, courtesy of* the Consumers Institute.

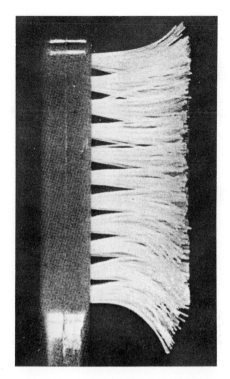

You should replace your toothbrush every two months or sooner – certainly before it starts to look like this.

How do you get rid of plaque?

This advice is from a Health Department leaflet.

The following dental cleaning aids will help you to remove plaque and keep your mouth healthy. Your dentist or dental nurse will show you how to use them correctly.

Toothbrush

The recommended toothbrush has a straight handle with a small enough head to let you reach every tooth. The bristles are of even length and a soft to medium texture. When they fray or become bent the toothbrush needs replacing.

Fluoride toothpaste

A toothpaste containing fluoride is recommended as the fluoride helps to make the tooth surface more resistant to decay.

Dental floss

Dental floss is a nylon thread which may have a coating of wax. Dental floss can be used to clean between your teeth where the toothbrush cannot reach but it is important for your dentist or dental nurse to show you how to use it before trying this yourself.

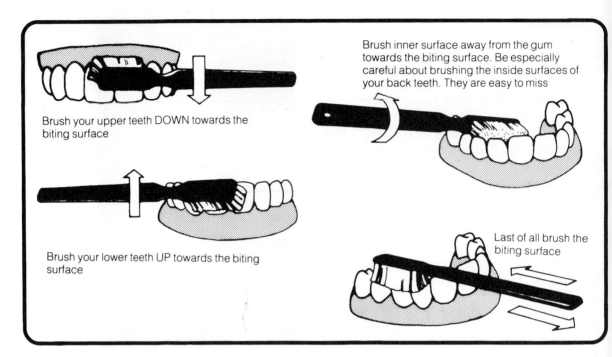

Brush your upper teeth DOWN towards the biting surface

Brush inner surface away from the gum towards the biting surface. Be especially careful about brushing the inside surfaces of your back teeth. They are easy to miss

Brush your lower teeth UP towards the biting surface

Last of all brush the biting surface

Brushing bonus

How to brush:
- Brush gently
- Brush away from your gums, but gently brush gums too—this will massage them.

What does toothpaste do?
- Toothpaste makes your mouth feel fresh.
- The brushing and flossing, not the toothpaste, remove plaque, though fluoride in toothpaste helps to toughen teeth and make them more resistant to decay.

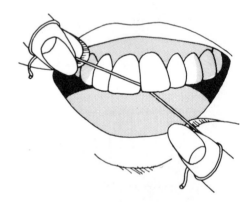

Dental floss

Floss your teeth once a day. Beat plaque (and decay, gum disease, bad breath). Buy waxed or unwaxed dental floss from the chemist.

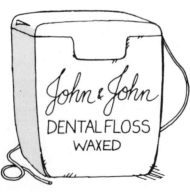

Watch your diet!

Here's more advice from a Health Department leaflet:

Does it matter what we eat?

Yes! Sugar causes tooth decay

When you eat any food containing sugar the sugar in it is quickly turned into acid. It is this acid on the surface of the tooth that eats into tooth enamel.

Save sweetened foods for mealtimes

WHY? . . . every time you eat something sweet your teeth are attacked by acid. If you save sweetened foods for mealtimes and reduce the number of acid attacks, this lessens the risk of tooth decay.

If you are hungry between meals

CHOOSE . . . unsweetened food such as cheese, bread (without sweet spreads), potato crisps, fruit, nuts, carrot sticks, and so on.

There are some sugar-free snacks in the Activity section at the end of this chapter. Your figure as well as your teeth will appreciate this sort of change!

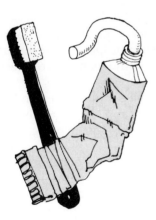

Toughening teeth

Fluoride toughens teeth and so helps prevent tooth decay. Drink fluoridated water or take fluoride tablets.

While your teeth are growing they absorb fluoride and build it right into their structure. Once they have stopped growing fluoride can still toughen teeth but only from the outside. The fluoride in fluoridated toothpaste toughens teeth from the outside too.

Visit your dentist

Dental care is free until you are 16 (or 18 if still at school). You will see the School Dentist occasionally and your own dentist regularly. They both want to help you keep your teeth and gums healthy. Modern equipment and methods mean that going to the dentist is not painful. Here are some of the things you gain by going to the dentist regularly:

Enjoyment of food

Most people like eating but the enjoyment can be spoiled by broken fillings or missing teeth. With sound teeth you can chew your food thoroughly and enjoy your meals.

Confident smile

Many careers are helped by a bright face, fresh breath, and a confident happy smile.

Happiness

Friendships can suffer if your teeth are dirty or neglected.

Good looks

To add to your personal confidence.

A healthy body and a feeling of well-being

Healthy teeth and gums are an essential part of feeling well and enjoying life.

Confidence to speak or sing

Teeth are essential for clear speech. Missing teeth can affect both speaking and singing.

Did You Know?

People who play contact sports know that wearing a mouthguard means they will save their teeth and their looks. You can buy mouthguards from the chemist or get one specially made for you by your dentist.

Hand-y hints

Think of all the things your hands do each day. They are the most important tools you have for work and leisure. But hands are more than tools. Like your face, your hands are always on show. People notice if they are dirty or damaged.

Wash hands:
- after going to the toilet
- before cooking or handling food
- after work
- after handling animals.

File nails smooth with an emery board or nail file—scissors can leave sharp edges.

If you run your finger nails over a cake of wet soap before you do dirty jobs like gardening, the dirt will wash out easily when you finish work.

Push the cuticles (skin around your nails) back gently after washing. Stops skin cracking, and look better too.

Clean nails with a nail brush, soap, and water. Never use metal instruments like scissors points. These roughen the nails and make them attract more dirt.

To protect the skin of your hands, you can:
- use a dishmop or brush when you wash up
- rub barrier cream into your hands before gardening, working on the bike, or washing dishes (barrier cream stops dirt and moisture from penetrating)
- take special care with sharp knives, graters, and tools
- use hand lotion or cream. Rub it into hands after you've washed or dried them
- use a pot holder or oven cloth to protect hands when using hot pots
- learn how to use tools and equipment, such as saws and motor mowers, safely.

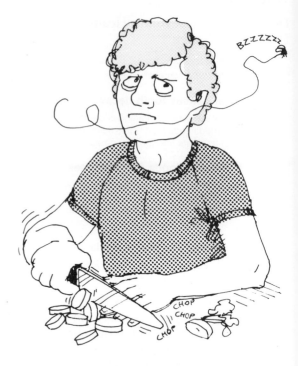

Off on the right foot

Feet have to carry the weight of your whole body. Feet need proper care or they may let you down. If your feet hurt, your face shows it!

Just how well people's feet stand up to a lifetime of wear and tear depends to a large extent on the shoes they wore as children and young adults.

Even before a baby is born the bones of its skeleton have begun to form. However many of them have not yet become the hard material that you would recognise as bone. They are made from a much softer material like the gristle you sometimes find in meat. This is called cartilage.

As the baby grows, more of this cartilage turns into hard bone. The bones of the baby's feet will go on growing until it is about eighteen years old! Until then, parts of them will be soft, and easily twisted out of shape.

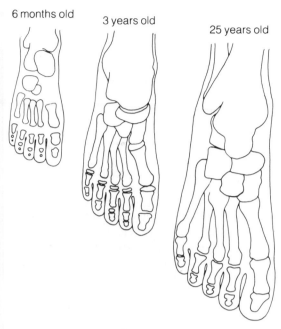

6 months old 3 years old 25 years old

How the bones in our feet grow

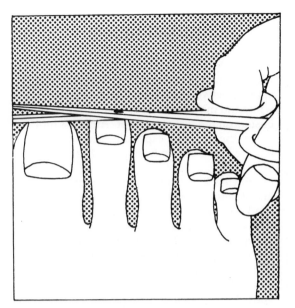

Cut toe nails straight across. It's very important to keep your toe nails trimmed when you go running

Shoes

Feet, especially ones which are still growing, need:

- growing room between toe and end of shoe
- firm fit at the heel
- enough width to allow for toe wriggling
- flexibility—to let foot muscles work
- a straight natural inner foot shape
- loose easy-fitting socks.

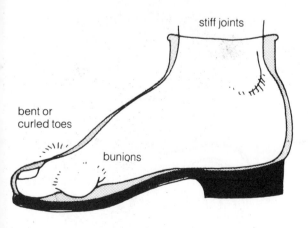

stiff joints

bent or
curled toes

bunions

The effects of poorly-fitting shoes

Foot care

The rules are simple:

- Wash feet often (at least once a day)
- Wear socks or tights which absorb sweat
- Change socks or tights every day
- Change shoes often! Air them when you're not wearing them
- Wash track shoes or sneakers inside and out regularly. Most sneakers can be washed in the washing machine
- Cut toe nails straight across to prevent them getting in-grown. In-grown toe nails are very painful
- Runners and joggers need to keep their toe nails cut short or they will get sore, turn black, and may even drop off
- If you have feet which sweat a lot, wear shoes made of material which 'breathes'. Wear cotton or wool socks as they absorb sweat best.

FOOTROT FAULTS

Athlete's foot

Athlete's foot is a **fungus** infection. It usually appears between the toes. The skin looks white and may be cracked. There may be tiny blisters on the rest of the foot. Athlete's foot makes the skin itch, especially when your feet are hot. Get help from your chemist, or your doctor.

Athlete's foot can happen to anyone—not just athletes. The fungus is picked up from dead skin on towels and clothes. (You may have white soggy skin between the toes if you are not careful enough about washing and drying your feet. This is not athlete's foot, and it will get better if you wash your feet daily, dry them carefully, and change your footwear regularly.)

Treatment: Ask the chemist for an ointment to kill off the fungus. If you get another attack ask your doctor for something stronger. Keep your feet cool, dry, and clean. Wash them every day and when they get hot after exercise. Dry them carefully especially between the toes. Then dust all over with talcum powder, but never use talcum on broken skin.

Socks or tights must be changed every day. It takes a bit of time and patience to get rid of athlete's foot.

Hint: Wear rubber sandals (flip-flops) right into the shower if you're staying in a hostel or on a campsite. Leave them on all through the shower and dry your feet carefully after. You won't get foot infections so easily.

Verrucae

Verrucae are warts which often appear on the foot, usually underneath. They may appear apart or in groups, and are often covered by hard skin. You may see brown and black dots on them. They can be very painful, especially when you pinch them. Verrucae are caused by a virus infection which can easily be picked up in swimming pools or in changing rooms.

Treatment: See your doctor.

Hard dry skin

Heels can get so dry in summer that they crack!

Treatment:
1 Soak your feet in soapy water. Rub the skin with pumice stone or a nail brush
2 Rub lanoline or vaseline into the dry parts. You can buy a cream especially for cracked heels from the chemist.

ACTIVITIES

Ears

1 Listen carefully for just five minutes. Write down *all* the sounds you hear. Now divide the sounds you heard into:
- sounds you like
- sounds you don't like
- noise you couldn't stand.

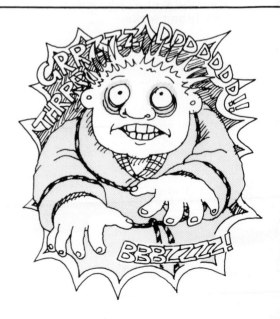

2 Write T (true) or F (false) next to the number of each statement, in your exercise book:

  1 sound is measured in decibels (dB)
  2 noise can damage hearing
  3 teenagers often have hearing loss
  4 a high decibel number means a loud noise
  5 sound travels in waves
  6 a loud noise makes your heart beat faster
  7 loud noise can cause pain
  8 another name for noise is 'unwanted sound'
  9 the world is noisier now than it was 50 years ago.

3 Discussion Questions:
* Why are you given a sweet to suck just before the aircraft lands?
* It is not a good idea to let a baby drink its bottle lying down. This can cause earache. Why?

4 Write down the good news about your ears and hearing.

All the statements in question 2 are true.

Eyes

1 Discuss how wearing a seat belt can protect your eyes.

2 Find out how to test for colour blindness.

3 Which eye care professional should these people go to?
(a) Auntie Beryl splashes neat bleach in her eyes
(b) Grandpa has broken his glasses
(c) Matthew squints
(d) Your friend can't read the sign on the front of the bus even when it is just stopping
(e) Tim is in the fifth form. He rubs his eyes a lot, especially after studying
(f) Tanya's eyes are glued up in the morning
(g) Greg is hit in the eye with a squash ball
(h) Your mum gets you to thread the needle for her.

Teeth

1 Find out what an orthodontist does.

2 *Mark the Plaque*
You will need a supply of disclosing tablets (or disclosing solution and cotton buds), available from dental supply firms, some chemists, or a dentist's surgery; dental floss; toothbrush and paste.

Half the class flosses between their top teeth. The other half of the class brushes their top teeth. Now use the disclosing tablets or solution, according to directions. Rinse mouths with water. Petroleum jelly on your lips will help prevent them becoming stained too!

On a copy of the tooth diagram below, each of you should colour in red where the dye has stained the plaque on your teeth.

Where is there most stain? (On which teeth, and where on the teeth?) Where does the plaque form most? Was there a difference between people who brushed and those who flossed?

3 In your exercise book write the good news about you and your teeth.

4 Make a low-sugar snack, in class or at home. Report on your success.

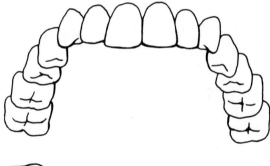

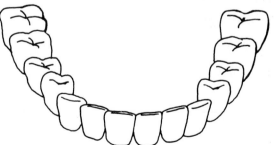

There are 32 teeth in a full set. Your set, like the one shown in the diagram, probably doesn't yet have the four 'wisdom' teeth—one at the back of each row

Low-sugar snacks

Bran Muffins (makes 12)

100 g plain flour
3 level teaspoons baking powder
50 g bran
1 level tablespoon sugar
1 egg
225 ml milk
2 tablespoons oil
4 dates, finely chopped
zest of an orange, finely grated

1. Turn oven on to 200°C (400°F), or gas mark 6.
2. Put the dry ingredients in a bowl.
3. Quickly stir in all the other ingredients.
4. Put the mixture into cake cases, making them two-thirds full.
5. Bake for 15 to 20 minutes.
6. Serve the muffins while they are still warm.

Roasted Peanuts

Spread raw peanuts in a roasting pan. Bake them in a moderate oven (180°C, or 350°F) for 15 minutes or until they are

- glistening with their own oil
- golden brown.

Check every few minutes to make sure they are not scorching. If you salt, sprinkle *very lightly* with garlic salt, onion salt, or celery salt. Drain on paper towels to absorb any extra oil.

Stuffed Celery

Fill a crisp piece of celery with cottage cheese mixed with chopped dried apricots, or dates, or chopped chives.

Yoghurt Banana Split

Fill peeled split banana with plain or flavoured yoghurt. Sprinkle with wheatgerm or shredded coconut and raisins.

Feet

1   Does your shoe fit?
(a) Draw around your shoe on paper.
(b) Take your shoe off and draw around your foot *over* the drawing of your shoe.
(c) How well does your shoe fit?
(d) Pin your outlines to a page in your exercise book.

2   Feel your foot while it is in its shoe. Does the shoe seem tight at any point on your foot when you walk? Can you wriggle your toes easily or are they nearly touching the end of the shoe? Does the side of the shoe press against your little toe?

If the answer to any of these is 'yes' the shoe is too small. (If the shoe slips on the heel or at the widest point of the foot, it is too large for you.)

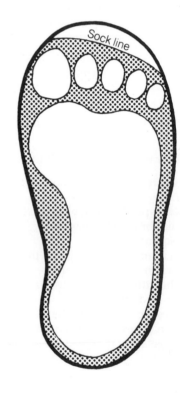

Hands

1 Reading with your hands.

Look at the table that shows the Braille alphabet of dots that blind people use. Now 'write' your first name in braille in your exercise book. Put each letter in a box as below. On the other side of the page, push the back of each dot of your braille writing with a pencil. Don't make a hole. Now feel the front side with your finger tips.

2 Discussion Questions:

How long should nails be? Why do netballers have a fingernail inspection before play begins? How can people stop biting their nails?

The Braille alphabet of dots

3
Keeping safe

Everyone wants to be healthy. But some people worry about their health too much. They

- fuss and worry about every little scratch or sniffle
- imagine they have serious illnesses or diseases
- think that to be healthy they have to take lots of pills and medicine
- visit the doctor for every little symptom.

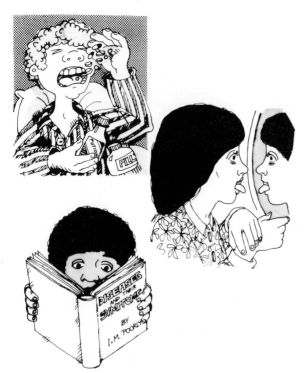

Other people are quite the opposite!

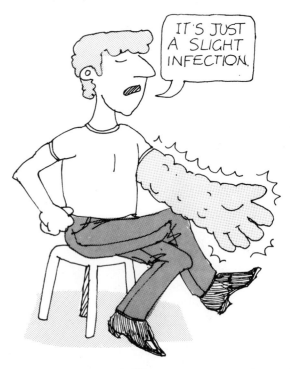

You should be sensible about your health. That is, you should make wise health choices, protect yourself from infections and injuries, not be over-anxious about yourself, or pretend you don't need help when you do.

Sometimes you may get ill or injured and need special health care. But it is best to stop things going wrong in the first place, if you can.

Prevention is better than cure!

There are obviously some things that *can't* be prevented, like:

- being knocked over on a pedestrian crossing
- catching a virus disease like chicken pox or mumps
- birth defects such as cleft palate
- getting acne at adolescence

but many other conditions *can* be prevented by making **sensible health choices**. For example,

- you are highly unlikely to get lung cancer if you don't smoke
- you are unlikely to get a liver disease called cirrhosis if you don't drink alcohol
- you won't get overweight if you eat the right amount of food for your height and energy requirements
- you won't injure your back if you lift heavy things properly
- you won't get athlete's foot if you care for your feet properly
- you are less likely to injure yourself if you get enough sleep
- you are unlikely to get rickets if you sunbathe.

Good hygiene will also help you to stay healthy.

- Food poisoning can be prevented by clean hands and utensils, and the proper heating, cooling, and storage of food.
- Many skin infections, like scabies, are unlikely where people are careful about washing their bodies and clothes.
- Wounds won't get infected if they are carefully cleaned and dressed.
- The spread of colds can be reduced if people keep their colds at home.
- People travelling overseas can avoid getting 'traveller's tummy' by drinking only bottled water, or water from a safe supply.
- Some forms of hepatitis can be prevented by careful hand-washing.

Medication, properly used, is an important aid to health:

- Diabetics protect themselves from diabetic coma by taking insulin
- Asthmatics can prevent attacks by using inhalers and other medication
- Epileptics control fits by taking the prescribed pills
- Alcoholics help themselves not to drink by taking 'Antabuse'
- People who are depressed can lead a normal life by taking anti-depressants
- Allergic reactions are reversed with anti-histamines
- Motion sickness (in cars, planes) can be prevented by pills.

Immunisation stops you getting sick in the first place!

- Young babies are immunised against diphtheria, whooping cough, tetanus, poliomyelitis and measles.
- Teenage girls are injected against German measles (rubella).
- All school pupils are immunised against TB (tuberculosis) as necessary.
- Overseas travellers may have to be inoculated against diseases like cholera.
- Some people are immunised against influenza.

Everyone has some control over his or her own health. As you get older you have to take more responsibility for keeping yourself safe. You have to prevent yourself from becoming ill or hurt. You also have to take some responsibility for other people—your family, friends, or others in the community.

CASE STUDIES

Health and Responsibility

Hugh had a party for his friends. They all liked cold chicken. He cooked it the day before and left it to cool in the kitchen. A few hours after the party all Hugh's friends, and Hugh too, were vomiting. They had food poisoning.

Robbie had four drinks on an empty stomach. On the way home he knocked down a pedestrian. She was taken to hospital with a cracked pelvis. Robbie lost his licence. He is still paying off the damage to the car, because his insurance policy didn't cover accidents where alcohol was involved.

Gina thought she'd had an immunisation against Rubella. But when Christopher was born he was blind. The doctors confirmed that Gina had had German measles early in her pregnancy.

At the Guy Fawkes party some of the kids were fooling around. Jeff threw a banger and it hit Emma and burnt her. She's embarrassed by the scar.

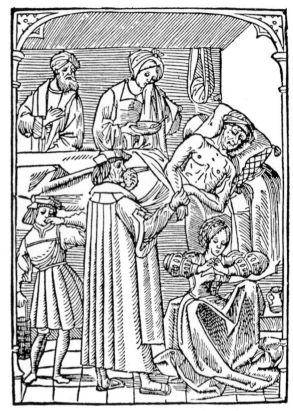

This old woodcut shows a doctor (sniffing a sponge soaked in rose-perfumed vinegar) and his assistant (holding his nose!) at a patient's bedside. For hundreds of years it was believed that bad smells transmitted diseases. Now we know that diseases like malaria (which is Italian for *bad air*) are in fact caused by living organisms invading our bodies

You will know of other cases where people have hurt others. Most *accidents* can be prevented by people being sensible, but we can't prevent all *diseases*, even though we may know what causes most of them.

People used to think that disease could be caught from bad air! They didn't realise that some diseases were contagious, and were spread by their own bad hygiene. Some societies even threw their garbage and body wastes into the street. No wonder people caught diseases such as Plague. Even in hospitals medical staff did not know the importance of cleanliness. Last century hospitals were very dirty indeed. Patients often died from an infection caught in the hospital rather than their own condition.

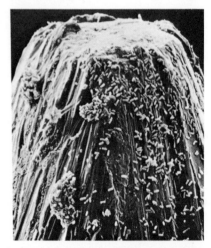

Magnified 500 times, the rod-shaped bacteria on the point of this pin are just visible   *Photo Dr Tony Brain, Science Photo Library Ltd*

How is disease caused?

Nowadays we know the causes of contagious diseases. We know that they are caused by micro-organisms—bacteria, fungi, or viruses. Sometimes people call all these micro-organisms 'germs'. Micro-organisms are in the air, in water, food, and on everything you touch. They are usually no problem because your body has defences against them—fine hairs in your nose, mucous lining to your nose and throat, acid in your stomach, unbroken skin, and white blood cells. It is only when micro-organisms get past your body's defences and multiply rapidly that a disease may develop.

The chart below shows the different diseases which bacteria and viruses cause. (Fungi are not so serious. They cause athlete's foot, ringworm, and thrush, and can be killed by fungicides in ointment or tablet form.)

	Bacteria	Viruses
Description	Very tiny. About a million cover a pin head	Only visible under an electron microscope. One million would fit inside *one* bacterium!
Where they live	Outside body cells where it is warm and moist, and there is food. Produce toxins (poisons)	Inside body cells. They change the working of the cells
Effect of antibiotics	Most bacteria are killed by antibiotics. (Some strains have developed a resistance to antibiotics)	Antibiotics have no effect on viruses
Some diseases they cause	sore throat food poisoning whooping cough pneumonia boils impetigo tetanus* typhoid venereal diseases	chicken pox herpes flu measles mumps polio rubella colds

* Everyone needs to be protected against tetanus. Everyone needs regular booster shots. Check yours.

Everyone knows that when a person is ill with a contagious disease it is easy to pass the sickness to another person, but even if you don't feel ill you can still spread disease, as a **carrier.**

How are diseases spread?

	How diseases are spread	Some of the diseases
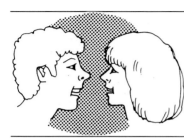	Moisture and mucus from nose, throat, and mouth: • sneezing • coughing • kissing • sharing things which others have had in their mouth • spitting	Colds, throat infections, measles, mumps, flu, glandular fever, tuberculosis, herpes simplex (cold sores)
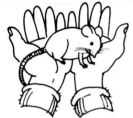	Hands not washed: • after going to the toilet (or changing babies' nappies) • before handling food, cooking food, or eating food • after handling pets or other animals	food poisoning diarrhoea vomiting dysentery hydatids (cysts produced by tapeworms) toxoplasmosis
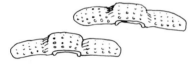	Open sores contain germs that are spread to other people	impetigo staphylococcal food poisoning boils

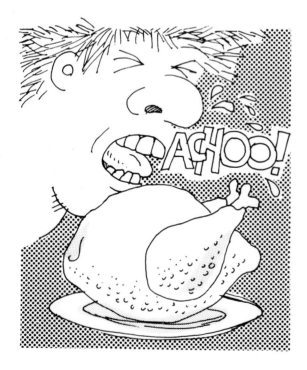

Many, many millions of germs live on you and every other human being. They cover your skin, hair and eyebrows, and congregate in folds and crevices. They live in your mouth, nose and throat, and nearly every body organ. In fact there are more bacteria living in your bowel than there are cells in your body! Of course most of these are harmless. Some do a useful job by producing vitamin K and some B vitamins.

> The danger is when bacteria from one part of you get into the other end of you!

Bacteria from your lower bowel can get into your mouth if you forget to wash your hands after you've been to the toilet. There will be bacteria on the toilet seat, on underpants, on skin. Toilet paper is no barrier to bacteria.

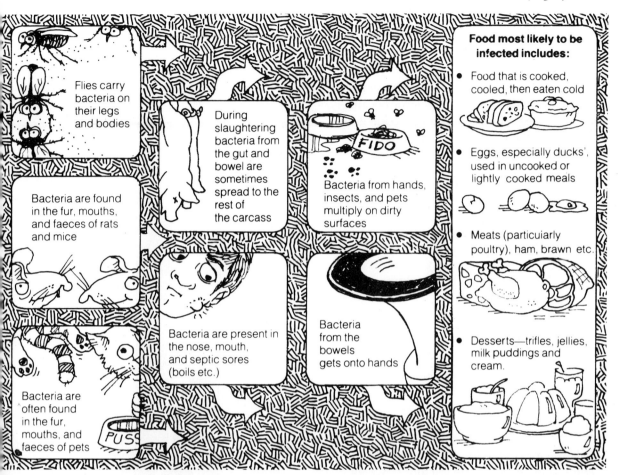

How bacteria get on to food

These bacteria can cause vomiting and diarrhoea.

Herpes simplex is a virus which causes cold sores around lips and mouth. But it is far more serious if it is transferred to the genitals, causing painful sores and blisters.

Children often transfer threadworms by scratching their bottoms. The threadworm eggs get under fingernails and re-infect the child when it puts food in its mouth. Of course threadworms aren't bacteria, but you can see how easily disease can be spread.

Keep your germs to yourself!

Germs can live and travel in food and water and on other things around the house like toothbrushes, bath towels and face cloths, cutlery, dish cloths, tea towels, bed clothes, and toys. Don't share germs! Follow these simple rules.

1 Use a tissue or handkerchief to cover sneezes and coughs. Dispose of tissues by flushing them away or burning. Stay at home if you have a cold.

2 Keep hands away from eyes, mouth, and nose.

3 Wash your hands with warm water and soap every time you go to the toilet, before you handle or eat food, and after handling pets.

4 Wash dishes in the hottest water you can. Dishwashers are very hygienic because the water can be hot enough to kill germs. Wash tea towels every day. Dish cloths can be soaked in bleach often. Bleach has a disinfectant action.

5 Keep hair, skin, and fingernails clean.

6 Don't share personal things. Keep your own combs, towels, face cloths, and toothbrush. Never wash these or yourself or your clothes in the kitchen sink.

7 Change clothes regularly so germs are killed by hot water, by sunshine, and by ironing.

8 Keep your house clean and aired out. This means your own room too.

9 Use the toilet brush for cleaning the toilet.

10 Handle food safely. You need to know some facts about food poisoning.

Food poisoning

Bacteria that cause food poisoning are commonly found in the gut and bowel of humans and animals, in sores, and in everyone's nose and throat. Bacteria can't move by themselves but cling onto anything that touches them, like hands, skin, clothes, or hair. Bacteria in the nose and throat are sprayed into the air when a person coughs or sneezes.

Bacteria are *everywhere:*

- in the air
- on our food
- on our hands
- on our cooking utensils . . .

. . . but this normally doesn't matter. Our bodies can usually cope with bacteria. There is danger only when bacteria **multiply.**

Millions of bacteria are needed to cause food poisoning. And with **time, warmth,** and **moisture** a few bacteria can multiply into millions.

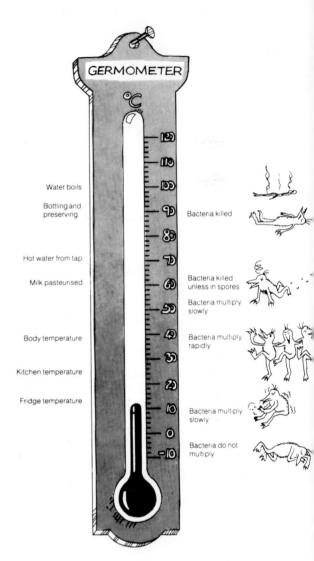

To be safe from food-poisoning bacteria you must be CLEAN, have hot food HOT, and cold food COLD. Why? because bacteria thrive on warm temperatures. They are killed at high temperatures. They are inactivated (stopped from multiplying) by low temperatures.

Cooking kills bacteria in food. If you eat it straight away—no danger. If you cool it quickly and keep it cold in the fridge, bacteria that have landed on it won't multiply so there's no danger. If you let food cool down slowly or leave it on the kitchen work top such bacteria will multiply rapidly. You are likely to be ill some hours after eating the food.

People often think they have 'stomach flu' or 'summer sickness' but really they are suffering from food poisoning. After reading all that about food poisoning and proper temperatures you may think that you are safe enough.

But there are some more dangers. As you know, freezing stops bacteria from multiplying. But it does not kill them. When frozen food is thawed the bacteria begin to multiply again. You must cook raw food that has been frozen, thoroughly.

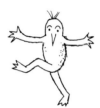

One germ

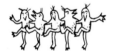

multiplies

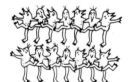

multiplies

multiplies

multiplies to
millions
in a few hours

Keep food cool

If you ever buy a cooked chicken that is still cold in the middle, or at all raw, *don't eat it*. If the shop or restaurant will not replace it, ring up the Environmental Health Office.

> Don't be satisfied with poor food care when you buy food or have a meal in a restaurant. As a consumer, your insistence in this matter is one of the most effective means of raising the standard of food care.
>
> Expect and ask for high standards from assistants serving food. When serving yourself use the tongs provided. Think of the people coming after you.
>
> Shop only in clean shops; refuse dirty service and explain why. Unsatisfactory food-servicing, food fingering, chipped or dirty dishes, should be drawn to the attention of the proprietor. You can feel confident that any offensive practice you notice is against Food Hygiene Regulations.
>
> You are also quite entitled and encouraged to bring such defects to the attention of your local Environmental Health Office.

Never be afraid to complain about food you find which is unsafe. It is your *right* to have safe food, and your *responsibility* to take action.

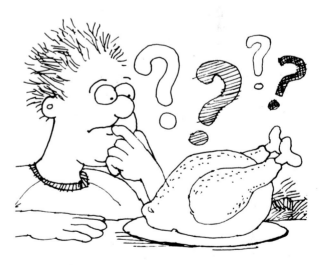

Magistrates order immediate closure of 'filthy' wine bar

AN EMERGENCY closure order has been imposed on a wine bar after maggots, larvae, mould and mice droppings were found during a spot check.

Magistrates imposed the order to "prevent danger to public health" despite hearing that the building was already closed for redecoration.

Health officers visiting the wine bar found decomposed food, smelly tea towels placed over food, a refrigerator virtually covered in mould growth and another with a foul-smelling liquid in the bottom, magistrates heard.

The court also heard the restaurant glasses and cutlery on the tables were dirty.

Health officer Mrs. Susan Smith said: "I certainly felt there was an imminent risk to the health of the public.

"I was immediately appalled when I saw the state of the kitchen. Everything seemed to be haphazard and muddled.

"I opened a refrigerator and found it was virtually covered in mould growth. There were pieces of mouldy cheese in the bottom of it. I noted that a lot of the equipment which would come into contact with food, such as pans and platters, were dirty and greasy. Many were encrusted with food debris."

Mrs. Smith said there was moulding and rotting food in the kitchen and a cucumber and grapes in a state of decomposition sitting in a foul-smelling liquor.

Shelves were dirty, so were containers, and there was no hot water serving the kitchen.

In the bar, she said, "I picked up some glasses and they were so dirty they were sticking to the plastic mat. I had to pull them off." In the storeroom she was confronted by maggots and hundreds of flies.

"In the corner on the floor there were bags and items of food stuffs. When I moved these, hundreds of fruit flies flew out at me. There were areas of maggots near the door, larvae of insects and mice droppings."

Mrs. Smith said that when she finished her visit members of the public were starting to go into the bar.

What signs might the customers have spotted that this wine bar was not a good place to eat?

ACTIVITIES

1 Which of these diseases or conditions could have been prevented? Which are beyond the person's control?

sunburn
mumps
flu
pneumonia
chapped lips
sprained ankle
blisters
smoker's cough
windburn
rubella
skin cancer
genital herpes

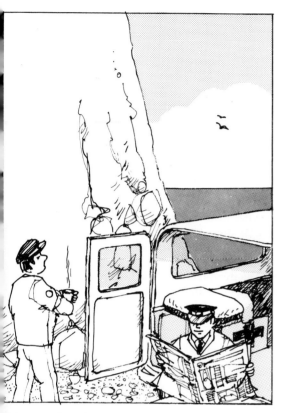

A tonne of cure!

2 'A fence at the top of the cliff is better than an ambulance at the bottom.' What does this mean?

3 A Health Education Council pamphlet about German measles (Rubella) begins:

**IS YOUR DAUGHTER
BETWEEN 11 & 14?**

Only teenage girls are immunised against Rubella. Is this the best way to eliminate the disease, and the risk it causes to unborn babies?

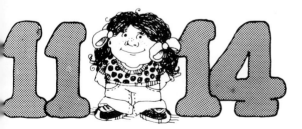

4 Only ⅕ of children in the developing world are immunised against measles, TB, tetanus, diphtheria, polio and whooping cough. 100% of children were vaccinated against polio and tetanus in the East Hertfordshire Health District. Try to explain this big difference and its likely effects.

5 Find out what insurance companies' policies are with
  drunken drivers
  young drivers
  unlicenced drivers.
Would the insurance company pay out if any of those people had an accident?

6 (a) Ask if your local Health Visitor, or a doctor, can come and talk to the class about preventing the spread of disease in the community, especially among teenagers.
(b) Check up on your tetanus shots. Are you due for a booster?

7 *First Aid*
Find out the best treatment and any preventive steps for the conditions below.
  Work out the ways you will find the information and record it. You will need to ask experts and use reference material. (The School Matron, the Health Visitor, the local pharmacy, doctors, Red Cross, St John's Ambulance may all be helpful.)
  bee stings (and wasp stings)
  insect bites
  burns
  cuts and grazes
  sunburn
  styes
  nosebleeds
  blisters

8 Arrange for class members to go for Red Cross First Aid Certificates.
List the things in an ideal first aid kit
(a) at home
(b) in the car.

9 Why don't doctors prescribe antibiotics if you have a bad cold with no other symptoms?

10 Find out the best home treatments for
  coughs and colds and flu
  sore throats
  diarrhoea and vomiting
  earache
  boils
  bruises
What signs would make you call the doctor?

11   The Royal Society for the Prevention of Accidents (RoSPA) runs many campaigns to prevent people being injured. Look at some of their leaflets, and find out what else RoSPA does.

Design a poster or pamphlet showing people how to lift heavy objects so they don't hurt their backs.

12   Injury is less likely if people know how to fall. Phys Ed teachers can show you these safe ways.

13   Do a project on one of these topics:
(a)   Find out about conditions in hospitals 100 years ago.
(b)   Who was Joseph Lister?
                  Louis Pasteur?
                  Edward Jenner?
(c)   In olden times (Middle Ages) what did people believe about the spread of disease?

14   It is important that separate knives or cutting machines are used for cooked and raw meats. This means either separate knives must be used, or knives must be washed in hot soapy water before cooked meat is cut. Why?

Is it safe for butchers to keep their knives in a holder around their waists? Why? Why not?

15   Is there danger in these situations?
(a)   Mince is cooked and eaten straight away.
(b)   Frozen hamburgers cooked on the barbecue are still red in the middle.
(c)   Bought meat pies are kept in the food warmer all day.
(d)   Cooked ham is left to cool in the cooking water overnight.
(e)   Cooked corned beef is cooled in the fridge.
(f)   Sam sneezes on raw meat.
(g)   Sam sneezes on cooked meat.
(h)   Fried chicken from the takeaway is pink in the middle.

16   What would **you** do?
Role play these situations:
(a)   You find that all the serving tongs are dirty at the sandwich bar
(b)   The person before you licks his fingers, picks up a paper bag and puts bread rolls into it, another person fingers two cakes before picking up one
(c)   You get a meal in a restaurant with a fly on the plate
(d)   There's glass in your bag of potato crisps.

17   What are the most important things you have discovered in this chapter?

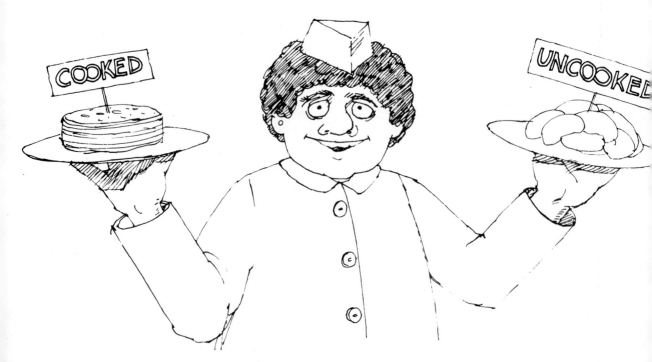

4
Eating—to enjoy, every day, everywhere

Do you want to
- look your best
- have plenty of energy for work and play
- do well at sport
- improve your fitness
- get strong
- be the right weight
- feel fine?

Then the food you choose is important for you.

People sometimes say 'You are what you eat.' This means that if you choose to eat sensibly you *can* be the way you want to. But it also means if you *don't* eat sensibly you may be

tired
the wrong weight
and not feeling at all well.

All right, you want to eat well—but it's hard to know just what that means. To see how much you know about food already, answer this quick quiz.

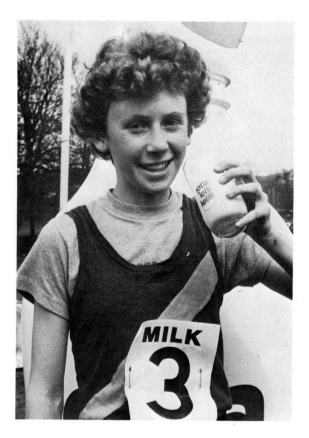

Quick Food Quiz

Write the numbers 1–20 in your book. Now write T (true) or F (false) alongside each question's number.

1 As your body changes you need to change your eating.
2 Taking vitamin tablets can make you ill.
3 Chocolate is bad for your skin.
4 You will lose weight if you eat less food than you use up as energy.
5 You don't need fibre in food.
6 Bread is fattening.
7 You need glucose for energy.
8 You can be healthy on a diet without meat.

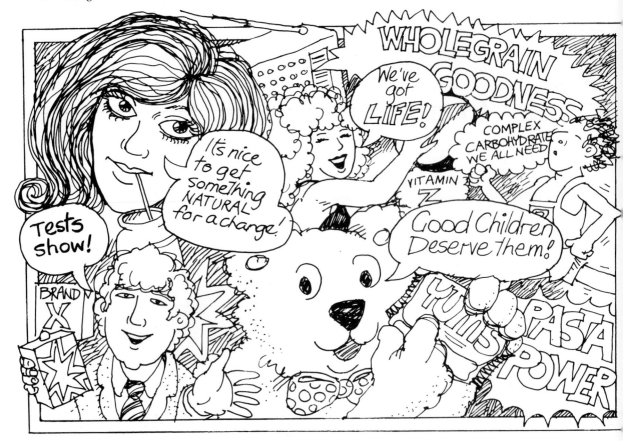

Media messages about food

9 Some foods are bad for you.

10 You are made up of what you eat.

11 You can buy health in a health food shop.

12 You should always be wary of a diet which contains just a few foods.

13 You can improve the way you feel, your fitness, and your looks by sensible eating.

14 People who live life to the full need diet supplements.

15 'Drinking fruit juice has got to be good for you.'

16 Natural vitamins are better than factory-made vitamins.

17 Eating extra salt with food can lead to high blood pressure.

18 Because it is grown without chemicals, organic food is better.

19 Grapefruit is slimming and 'melts fat away'.

20 Drinking water is good for you.

Find the answers on page 46 in this chapter. In your exercise book, circle the answers you were surprised at.

You hear and see a lot of information about food, drinks, eating, and diet. How do you know

- what to eat
- if some foods are 'good'
- if there are really 'bad' foods
- what makes you fat
- what you need
- how to make good choices?

It is very confusing. There are so many different messages about food and health—messages in magazines, newspapers, and on the radio and TV—from people who want to sell food. Some messages may be true and some may be partly true. But others may be quite misleading. How do **you** know which are the right messages? To understand messages you need to know some Facts.

Food Facts

All foods are made up of useful ingredients, called **nutrients**. The nutrients' names are:

Carbohydrates (Sugar and Starches)
Proteins
Fats (and Oils)
Minerals
Vitamins
Water.

Nutrients are important. You often read about them in magazines. Or you see them on TV or hear about them on the radio. People have even written whole books about nutrients.

Food has different jobs to do in your body (and everyone else's too, of course). Food is for Growth, and Repairing, as well as for Energy. Some of the nutrients in food are used by your body for Growth and Repair. Some of the nutrients are used by your body for Energy.

You never see a menu like this:

Menu

Calcium Cocktail
Vitamin E Entrée

Grilled Carbohydrates
Mashed Protein
Pan-cooked minerals

Vitamin C Custard
Frozen Fat

This is because people eat *food*, not *nutrients*. Nutrients are part of all foods.

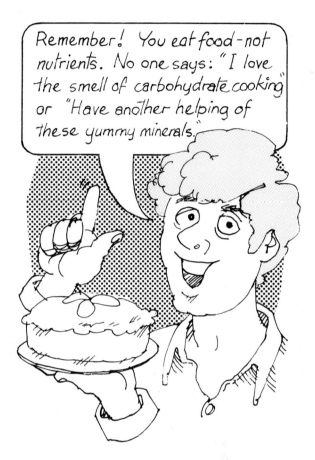

Remember! You eat food - not nutrients. No one says: "I love the smell of carbohydrate cooking" or "Have another helping of these yummy minerals."

All foods (except sugar and oil) are made up of **mixtures of nutrients**. So all foods (except sugar and oil) provide nutrients for all body processes.

No one food is essential for growth. You need a variety of foods for growth.

No one food is essential for energy. You need a variety of foods for energy.

Nutrients	Uses
The nutrients your body uses for GROWTH are • proteins • some minerals • some vitamins • water	You grow taller and larger Fingernails grow Hair grows
Your body uses the same nutrients for REPAIRING itself as for growth	Wounds heal Broken bones mend New skin replaces worn-off skin
The nutrients your body uses for ENERGY are • carbohydrates (both sugars and starches) • fats and oils • other minerals • other vitamins • water	You need energy to **keep alive**— your heart beats your lungs breathe your brain thinks —to **keep warm**, and to **be active**: do work play sports move about

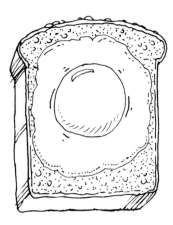

Total weight: 75 g
kJ: 780
Protein: 10 g
Fat: 8.5 g
Carbohydrate: 13 g
Vitamins & Minerals: 1 g
Fibre: 1.5 g

Even a simple meal like this poached egg on buttered toast provides a variety of nutrients. Why do you think the food weighs about 40 g more than the nutrients it contains?

CASE STUDIES

Food Facts—Messages Muddled!

Lisa went to gym club. She begged her mother to buy a certain fruit biscuit because the TV ad said 'how can you do without them?' and showed a girl eating some biscuits and doing gym exercises perfectly.

Elena always felt tired. She went to the chemist and bought multi-vitamin tablets. She thought she would feel better.

Ross was training for athletics. He had heard a well-known athlete say that you need glucose for instant energy. Ross was disappointed to find that his time was just the same, even when he took the glucose just before his race. Then he took special drinks. They didn't work either.

Brendon's mum read about a high-fibre slimming diet. She decided to sprinkle bran on all her food. She had **fibre** with everything. Brendon's mum felt really awful for days . . .

Danny thought he would grow more if he always had a certain cereal for breakfast: 'Milko today builds champions of tomorrow.'

There are no magic foods. There is no magic formula. There probably never will be!

What to eat and how much to eat and drink still causes arguments among doctors, scientists, and even family members.

Scientists, doctors, nutrition experts, and dietitians *do* agree on two things:

Agreement 1 There is still a lot to learn about food. New research is going on all the time. Nobody knows everything about healthy eating. Be suspicious of advice that says you *must* eat 'such and such' or you must have a certain amount of it, or that you must *not* eat so-and-so.

Agreement 2 Many people become ill or die before they should because of the way they eat or used to eat. Their **diet*** has affected their health.

So the experts give two pieces of advice:

Advice 1 Eat a wide variety of food (eat many different foods in your diet). This means you have many kinds of food and drink, and also try new foods. Eating only a few kinds of foods is not sensible.

Advice 2 Try to follow the **National Guidelines** on nutrition in Britain. These are guidelines to help you eat sensibly and well.

1 *Eat a variety of foods each day.* (Sounds familiar? You can see how important variety is.) We need about 40 nutrients in different amounts to stay healthy. Eating a variety helps to make sure that you don't get too much or too little of any one nutrient.

2 *Eat only as much as you need.* One of the main problems people in developed countries face is being overweight. Overweight people feel miserable and get tired easily. They are often unhappy with their appearance and are more likely to get ill.

3 *Eat less sugary food and more starchy food.* Starchy foods like bread, cereal, and potatoes are satisfying and filling. They also give you plenty of fibre for their weight. Sugary foods are very high in energy for their bulk and also cause tooth decay.

4 *Eat less fat.* You can do this by cutting fat off your meat, spreading butter thinly, and cutting down on fried foods.

5 *Eat less animal food.* Have smaller helpings of meat, cheese, and dairy products. Have larger helpings of **cereals**, thicker slices of bread, more rice, and more **legumes** such as dried peas and beans and lentils.

6 *Use less salt.* Go easy on salt. Put less in cooking and don't sprinkle it on food when you eat it. You won't miss it after a while. Make sure the salt you do use is iodised.

7 *Increase the amount of dietary fibre in your diet.* Experts believe that fibre is needed for your digestive system to work well. It speeds up the passage of food wastes and prevents constipation.

8 *Drink less alcohol.* Beer, wine, and spirits are all high in energy, so they can make you put on weight. People who drink a lot may not have good eating habits and can get quite sick. New evidence shows that even a small amount of alcohol can harm an unborn baby. Australia's Nutrition Guidelines say 'enjoy drinking water'.

9 *Use fluoridated water* to cut down on tooth decay.

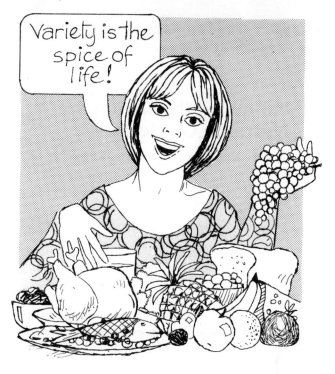

Variety is the spice of life!

---

* Diet? Everyone is on a diet. A diet is a person's usual food *not* special food for slimming.

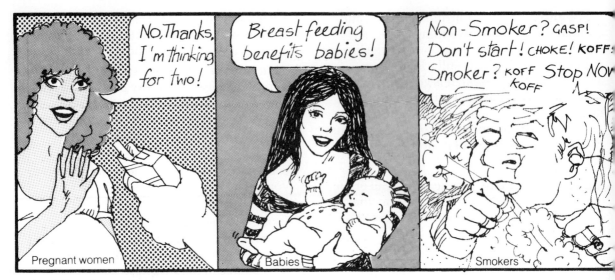

Guidelines for special groups

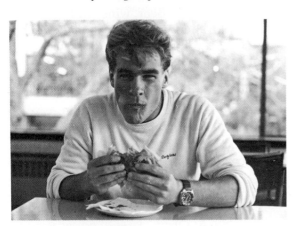

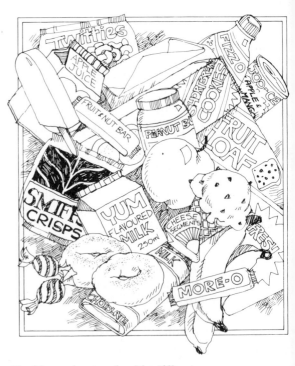

Healthy and not-so-healthy 'fillers'

Following the National Nutrition Guidelines

Choose and eat meals and snacks like these every day:

- plenty of bread, potato, rice, or pasta
- plenty of fruit and vegetables
- a bit of fish, chicken, eggs, cheese, or meat (beef, mutton, or pork).

Eating like this is easy! It just means a few changes. Start at the beginning—start with breakfast. Eat something before you leave home in the morning. You can eat a little or a lot. It depends on how hungry you are, and how much time you have. If you are hungry,

eat lots and lots! If you aren't at all hungry, have a snack because it is probably at least 10 hours since your last meal. You have digested all of that meal so you need some food, first thing. Everyone can find something to eat in the cupboard or fridge.

(There are some **breakfast recipes** in the Activity section at the end of this chapter.)

Breakfast

No time to eat?	A bit of time?	More time? (& hungrier?)
Pick up either: • a sandwich—make it with thick bread, a bit of butter and any filling • a banana and some milk • a piece of bread pudding • some fruit • a cold sausage	Fix either: • cereal and milk • muesli and yoghurt • toast and low fat spread • toasted muffins • cheese on toast • banana milkshake • milk drink	Cook either: • porridge and milk • french toast (non-stick frying pan) • eggs on your toast (occasionally) • some baked beans, or spaghetti or sweet corn • tomato on toast

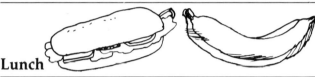 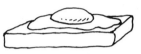

Lunch

Lunch from Home?	Buying Your Lunch?	Lunch at Home?
Pack up either: • sandwiches or bread rolls with any filling you like, some fruit • scones or muffins • boiled egg or cold meat with your sandwiches • raisins and cheese segments • leftovers! • salad • soup in a vacuum flask	Choose either: • sandwiches or rolls • soup and buns • hamburger or pizza • pies, fish and chips, fried chicken, and hot dogs are fine, BUT once or twice a week is enough • buy some fruit if you can • choose fruit juice rather than fizzy drink	Make either: • dishes made from bread, or pasta, rice, potatoes with some egg, fish, meat, or cheese • hot American sandwiches • toasted sandwiches • open sandwiches • salad • soups • mini pizzas • pizza

Lunch recipes: For mini pizzas, open sandwiches, hot American sandwiches (as well as fillings ideas for ordinary sandwiches), see the Activity section at the end of this chapter.

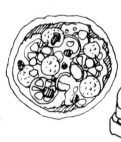 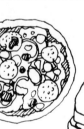 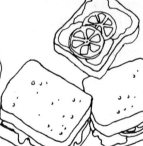 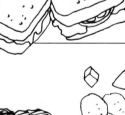

Dinner

Eat:
• a smaller helping of meat—choose lean meat
• plenty of potato or rice or pasta or noodles
• plenty of other vegetables
• fruit puddings or fruit or crackers and a bit of cheese for after.
Try not to add extra salt or sugar to your food.

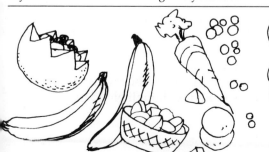 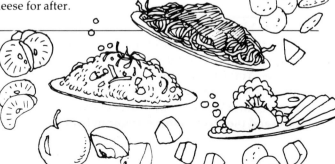 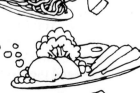

Snacks and Drinks

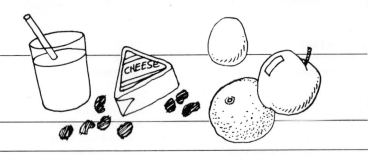

Look for snacks which are:
- good for your shape
- kind to your teeth
- in line with the nutrition goals.

Athlete's Additions	Body Builder's Bonus	Slimmer's Summary

Follow the Nutrition Guidelines. No special extras are needed. You'll get all the foods you need for performance from eating this way.
 	
    People doing long distance running need to eat extra starches like bread and potatoes.
	Follow the Nutrition Guidelines. Eat more snacks: milk-drinks, yoghurt, cheese, nuts, sandwiches, rolls.	Follow the Nutrition Guidelines. Cut back on sweets, butter, margarine, cream, fried foods. Use non-fat or skim milk.
		
		    More for you in Chapter 5: **Eating Safely.**

Answers to the Quick Food Quiz

1   True.
2   True. Certain vitamins can be stored by the body. Vitamins A, D, and E are like this. If you take too much of these fat-soluble vitamins you can get very ill. Never take vitamin tablets unless you've asked your doctor. Any extra water-soluble vitamins (B and C) are passed out in your urine.
3   True. There is no magic answer to skin problems but eating sensibly does help. Concentrate on plenty of fresh fruit and vegetables, whole grain bread and cereal. Some people may find that chocolate affects their skin.
4   True. This is the sensible way to weight loss.
5   False. Fibre in food helps to clear the body of waste, and prevents constipation. It sweeps the unwanted food along the intestine. You get fibre in plant foods from the cell walls. Too much fibre will give you wind.
6   False. Slimming diets should include some bread—if two or more slices are included you can be fairly sure it's a sensible diet.
7   False. You can get all the energy you need without ever eating sugar bowl sugar or glucose. There's energy in nearly every food—and plenty of natural sugar in fruits.

What's more, you can absorb the sugar from an orange through your stomach into the bloodstream in just 4 minutes. Glucose is simply an expensive form of sugar.
8   True. Other foods can replace meat.
9   False. No one food is 'bad' for you. However eating too much of one food can mean others get left out.
10   True. Nothing else turns into you but food.
11   False. You can't buy 'health' anywhere—ordinary supermarkets are really your health food stores.
12   True. No one food can make you healthy. A good variety of food is important.
13   True.
14   False. People who live life to the full are people who eat sensibly and need no supplements.
15   False. Fruit juice is refreshing. It is good to enjoy fresh fruit, too—for the crunch and munch, and the fibre. Some canned juices have added sugar. All canned juices are quite high in energy.
16   False. Your body cannot tell the difference between vitamins that occur naturally in food and those that are factory made.
17   True. Researchers believe a high salt intake is linked with high blood pressure.

18 False (nearly always). The composition of a potato (or tomato or apple or whatever) grown with compost and the composition of a potato (or whatever) grown with chemical fertilisers are the same. Sometimes the chemicals used to kill pests cling to food and this may be dangerous to humans.

19 False. Like most fruits, grapefruit is low in energy value and high in fibre. But it has no special fat-melting properties.

20 True. Experts think it is good to drink water instead of high energy drinks like soft drinks and alcohol.

ACTIVITIES

1 In the table below, the nutrition goals and the *hows* and *whys* of reaching them have got mixed up. Sort them into three columns in your book so that they are clear and you have the *right* messages.

Goals	How?	Why?
1 Eat a variety of food	Don't think a day's food must have meat in it	Fluoride builds strong teeth and helps stop tooth decay
2 Increase fibre	Don't automatically use salt in cooking. Learn not to add salt to the food on your plate	Alcohol damages your body. Heavy drinking often means a poor diet
3 Eat less fat	Take tablets if your water is not fluoridated. Fluoride toothpaste toughens teeth too	Fibre helps get rid of wastes and keeps your bowels healthy
4 Eat less animal food (meat, etc.)	Eat many different foods, not a lot of a few foods	It is easy to eat too much sugar. This leads to excess weight and tooth decay
5 Eat less sugar (more starchy food)	Maintain normal weight. To lose weight decrease food intake and increase exercise	Animals foods are high in fat. Eating less of them cuts down on fat
6 Eat only as much as you need	Drink no more than two drinks (beer or wine or spirits) a day	Too much salt is associated with high blood pressure
7 Use fluoridated water if you can	Cut down on fried foods. Cut fat off meat. Spread butter or margarine more thinly	Your body will get everything it needs
8 Use less salt	Bulky, starchy foods like bread, potatoes, baked beans, and cereals have lots of fibre	Overweight people get more diseases and die earlier
9 Drink less alcohol	Eat less cakes, biscuits, sweets, puddings, and fruit squash	Too much fat will make you overweight and may be one of the causes of heart disease

2 *Pick the pairs*

Here are some pairs of foods and meals. Which
one in each pair scores a goal? (A nutrition goal, of
course!) Copy the table below into your
exercise book. Tick one in each pair and say which
goal it scores, and why. The first one has been
done for you.

A	B	Why it wins	Goal No.
Iced raspberry bun	Plain currant bun ✓	It cuts down on sugary food—no icing	5
Meat pie, pastry topping	Meat pie, potato topping		
Raw peach	Tinned peach (in syrup)		
Strawberry flavoured and sweetened yoghurt	Plain yoghurt mixed with strawberry purée		
Fried steak and french fries (chips)	Spaghetti and meat sauce		
Honey Puffs and milk	Oatmeal porridge and milk		
Raw peanuts	Salted roasted peanuts		
Orange juice	Orange		
The Colonel's fried chicken	A hamburger		
Fresh fruit salad	Cheesecake with fruit topping		

Discussion questions

1 If you take any extra water-soluble vitamins
(the B group or vitamin C), the extra will be passed
out of your body in urine and flushed down the
toilet. (Remember that any extra of the fat-soluble
vitamins—Vitamin A, D, or E—is stored in the
body and can build up to poisonous levels.)

Mineral and Vitamin pills are widely advertised.
They suggest if you feel a bit
    'off-colour'
    'less than well'
    'poorly'
    'lacking in energy'
    'not your best'
that you should take some of their (expensive)
tablets and you will be on top of the world.

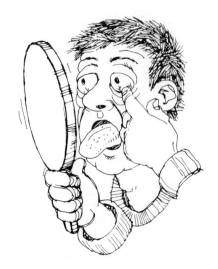

Someone once said, 'The Americans have the most expensive urine in the world.' Why is their urine expensive? Do we have expensive urine too?

2 People often *do* feel better after they have taken pills, even when the pills have no proven medical benefit. How can this be?

3 (a) What does this saying mean: 'She is digging her grave with her knife and fork'?
(b) What is dangerous about being overweight?

4 Suggest four ways to lower the amount of salt you eat.

5 Many of the eating habits we have now come from our farming background. We had generous meals with plenty of meat, butter, and eggs; we had big, hearty morning and afternoon teas of scones, pies, and cakes. How suitable are these meals for us today?

6 In groups make up a Nutrition Goals Game. It could be like the one illustrated, or like Snakes & Ladders or a 'question and answers' game.

7 Research nutritious lunch dishes. Find recipes for dishes based on bread, pasta, rice, or potato which include some egg, meat, fish, or cheese. Make them in class if you can.

8 Survey the foods that are sold in your school's canteen or tuck shop, or the snack and lunch foods sold at the shop nearest your school. Write a list in your book. Circle the foods which are the best choices for people who want to eat well and feel fine.

9 The table below shows how much of these foods we eat on average in Britain each week.

Food	Average amount per person per week
Milk	4 pints
Cheese	100 grams
Butter, margarine, lard, cooking fat	250 grams
Eggs	3–5 eggs
Sugar	250 grams
Beef, veal, lamb, pork, bacon, ham	500 grams
Poultry	175 grams
Offal	25 grams
Sausages	75 grams
Breakfast cereals	100 grams
Fish	125 grams
Fresh green vegetables	275 grams
Bread	775 grams

Discuss what this table tells you about our eating habits. Which of these things does it tell you?
(a) We choose lean foods instead of fatty ones.
(b) We eat a lot of sugar.
(c) We are sticking to the Nutrition Guidelines.
(d) We eat a lot of meat.
(e) We eat high fibre bread and breakfast cereals.
(f) We eat a lot of dairy foods.
(g) We all eat sausages.
(h) We spend more on poultry than on fish.
(i) Bread is an important part of our diet.
(j) We eat very little offal.
(k) More is spent on meat than on other foods.

Recipes

French Toast

2 eggs
2 tablespoons milk
4 slices bread
1 tablespoon butter

1. Beat the eggs and milk with a fork.
2. Dip the slices of bread into this mixture. The bread will soak up the egg mixture.
3. Melt half of the butter in a non-stick frying pan. When it sizzles, put in the bread.
4. Cook till golden, turn over and cook till second side is golden (add more butter if the first lot has gone).
5. Cut slices in half or cut in fingers. Serve at once on warmed plates, with a light sprinkling of sugar. Makes 8 pieces.

Ch'apple Toast

⅛ teaspoon dry mustard (if you like)
100 ml milk
½ cup (50 g) tasty cheese, grated
1 apple, chopped or grated (no need to peel)
4 slices hot buttered toast
pinch salt
shake pepper

1. Mix seasonings and milk well. Stir in the cheese and apple.
2. Spread on the toast. Bring the topping right up to the edge of the toast.
3. Put under a hot grill until bubbly.
4. Serves 4.

Open Sandwiches

On one layer of bread spread:
1. margarine, low fat spread, butter, cottage cheese, or mayonnaise
2. a layer of lettuce
3. a layer of thin-sliced cheese or meat, sausage, or ham
4. top with pineapple piece, lettuce, tomato, pickle, sliced hard-boiled egg, onion rings, cucumber, asparagus tips, spring onion, radish. (Try 2 or 3 of these.)

Use a toothpick to hold the topping on the bread if you like.

Sandwich Fillings

Marmite and chopped nuts
Salami and mustard
Ham and pineapple
Cream cheese and ginger or dates
Green peas and mint
Cheese and tomato
Cold meat and lettuce or pickle
Baked beans and grated cheese
Cheese and apple
Curried egg
Egg and watercress
Banana and lemon juice

Mini Pizzas

Halve a hamburger bun. Toast both halves. Spread with tomato puree, grated cheese. Sprinkle with these if you like:
● bits of ham or bacon
● basil or thyme or mixed herbs.
Grill until bubbly.

Hot American Sandwiches

Take some fairly thick slices of bread and toast one side of each slice. Spread the untoasted side thinly with butter, cottage cheese, or mayonnaise. Fill with a hot filling, like heated up:

    roast meat and gravy
    corned beef and mustard
    mince
    stew or casserole
    eggs—scrambled, boiled, or fried
    bacon—fried or grilled
    sliced ham
    fish—tinned or cooked

Top with salad vegetables.
Season with relish, pickle, chutney sauce, mustard, or mayonnaise.
Top with second slice of toasted bread, serve.

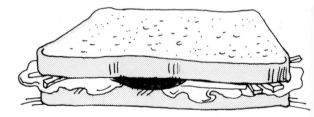

5
Eating safely

Can the food you eat do you harm? Yes! If you eat less than you need, or too much, it can harm you. (Food can also be harmful if it is contaminated by infection or poisonous substances.)

Getting the right amount of food

If you are getting just enough food your weight will be in proportion to your height. You will feel fit and fine. Your food intake and your activity will balance.

Balancing your activity and your food means that the energy you get from food and drink equals the energy you use up for keeping alive (the work of your body systems), keeping warm, and being active (work, play, and exercise). The energy in food is measured in kilojoules*, and the energy your body uses up is measured in kilojoules. Slight differences from day to day between the kilojoules you take in and the kilojoules you use up won't make a change in your weight. It is over a period of time that weight will change.

So losing weight means two things. It means eating less food and doing more exercise. Putting on weight means two things too! It means you have been eating more food and doing less exercise.

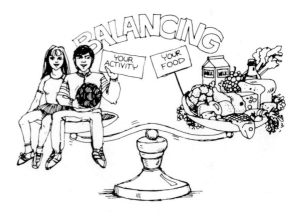

Most people in the UK are more concerned with losing weight. There is more about losing weight later in this chapter. But a few people, usually teenage girls, can't control their drive to lose weight. They have a disease called *Anorexia Nervosa*. Girls who have this disease see themselves as fatter and wider than they really are. They get more and more active, and exercise really hard! At the same time they are eating less and less. Some days they may eat nothing at all. Other times they eat but feel so guilty afterwards that they make themselves vomit.

---

*Kilojoules were once called Calories. If you find old Calories charts you can convert to kilojoules by multiplying by 4. This is a rough measure. For example:

80 Calories × 4 = 320 kJ

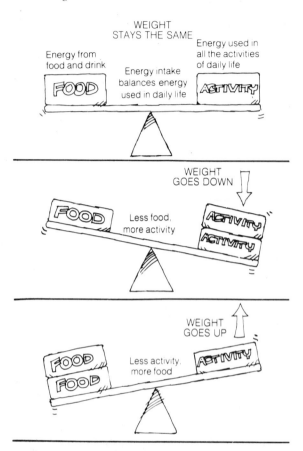

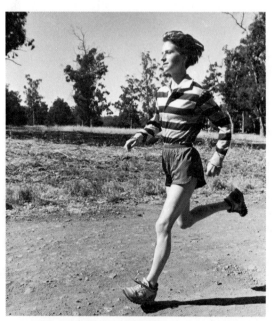

This girl is recovering from anorexia   *Photo by Jeff Reinking, reproduced courtesy* Runners World *Magazine*

Questions about Anorexia (The 'Skinny Disease')

Q: How can I tell the difference between a very thin person and a person who might have anorexia?

Mother

A: A girl with anorexia nervosa starts to look like a walking skeleton. She will lose her natural body curves and be very bony. She often wears a lot of clothes (this is because an anorexic is always cold) so you may not realise how very skinny she is getting. She will stop getting her monthly period. This is because her body's hormones are disturbed by her extreme weight loss. Other signs you could notice: she may become covered with long fine hairs, and she may lose hair from her scalp. It is possible that she will talk about food a lot and often 'take charge' of the kitchen at home.

Q: What do I do? I think my friend Jane has anorexia. She has lost 12 kilos this year and she looks awful. She says she's perfectly all right. I know her parents are worried . . .

Joe

A: Enlist the help of your School Matron. He or she is trained to help your friend. Girls with anorexia often resist their parents' suggestions that they see a doctor. They deny that there is anything wrong. This is probably because their image of their own body is distorted—a bit like looking in a mirror at the fun fair. Jane will probably need hospital treatment and a lot of help and support.

Q: My friend Stacy is 16. She is normal weight for her height. I know this because we get weighed at the gym. But sometimes she binges on food—just stuffs herself full. Then she goes and makes herself sick. Has she got the skinny disease?

Emily

A: It sounds as if Stacy has a similar disease. It is called *Bulimia*. This means that the person binges on enormous quantities of food and then gets rid of it—by vomiting or taking laxatives. Often the person seems successful at school or work but eats because of hidden stress in her life. She usually manages to keep herself at the right weight. A bulimic person is usually disgusted by her behaviour, so Stacy may need special help too.

Probably only about 1 girl in 100 will suffer from these eating diseases. Very few boys are affected—only about 5 per cent of sufferers are male. In fact, in Britain people are more likely to be overweight than underweight. Many fat people pretend to be happy. Even their friends don't know they are miserable underneath. But overweight people hide their true feelings. Some of them don't believe the scales, and they may have a distorted body image too.

Will you please publish this letter? I want other teenagers to know my story about anorexia and my struggle with starvation.

I felt powerful when I found out that I could lose weight better than anyone else. First I just ate cottage cheese, grapefruit and coffee – then I just nibbled raw vegetables. I started feeling that anything I ate would make me FAT. Soon I could go for three days without eating. I kept telling Mum I was O.K. Sometimes I'd eat a bit of dinner to please them but then. I found I could get rid of the horrible full feeling by making myself sick. I really resented my friends if they nagged me to eat. I knew I was getting thin, because the scales showed it. But my mind wouldn't believe it. I still felt FAT. I used to run for several hours a day, study hard, and get less sleep – sometimes only three hours. Not only did I run, but I ran with a vengeance. If I ate two carrots I'd have to run two km. to make sure I didn't gain a gram. Instead of strengthening my muscles, running was breaking them down. I began to faint and have dizzy spells. Mum took me to the doctor who said I was anorexic and put me in hospital.

That was two years ago. You know, I'll probably never be cured, but at least with treatment and counselling I am learning to eat properly. I feel better about myself and feel that I am in control of me – not just my eating...

Liane

CASE STUDIES

Facing the Fact of Fatness

Nani finally found enough courage to go to a weight watching group. She was 45 kilos overweight—that is nearly the weight of another person. She was shocked when the group leader came up to her and said, 'Have you come to join today?' Nani said to herself, 'How does she know I'm fat?'

Becky consoled herself with food. Whenever she felt tired, depressed, cross, let down, bored, or just miserable she would eat. She knew she was putting on too much weight and kept trying to find easy ways to lose it—crash diets, special drinks, and even sweets you sucked before a meal. Nothing worked for long. This depressed her so much she had to eat to cheer herself up!

George used to make everyone in the class laugh. He really played the fool, especially in P.E. All his jokes were about himself and his weight. The kids all liked him but he was never a member of any team.

A lot of people are fat for reasons we don't understand. One thing we do know is that practically no one can blame their 'glands'. Some experts believe that overfed babies will have weight problems later on.

Young teenagers may get a bit fat before they begin their growth spurt. But usually people are overweight because they have taken in more kilojoules in their food than they have used up in their physical activity, over a period of some years.

There is a solution. It is not a magic overnight cure—in spite of what the ads say.

The weight plan that works

To lose weight safely you need four things:

1 To take in less kilojoules in your food and drink. (The only liquids which give no kilojoules are water and black coffee or tea.)

2 To use up more kilojoules in your physical activity.

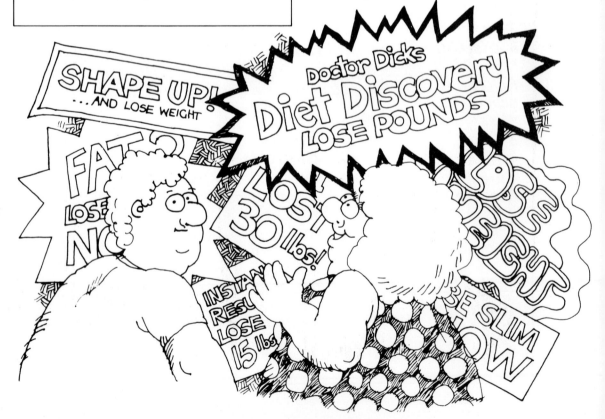

3 Time. It is not safe to lose more than 500–1000 g per week. The weight you lose in the first week is almost all water. Fast weight loss on a 'crash' diet is usually followed by fast weight gain back!

4 Knowledge. Slimming diets need to follow the nutritional goals too. You need to know which foods give you a lot of kilojoules and which activities use up a lot of kilojoules. You need to know that a diet is *your usual eating*, not something you do for a week or two.

The plans that *don't* work

Massage and Massage Belts

Massaging shakes or vibrates parts of your body. It can be relaxing but it won't move your fat off your body.

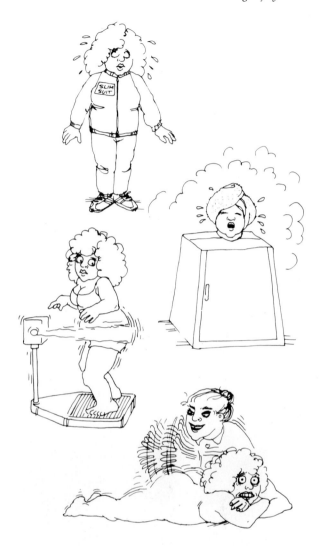

Rollers

These machines roll up and down on a body part like a rolling pin on dough. They do not remove fat or improve your appearance.

Electric currents

Machines that cause an electric current to go to a muscle and make it move can be dangerous to the heart and other internal organs and should not be used except by doctors or physiotherapists.

Plastic suits

Some people think plastic or rubberised suits are good to wear because they make you perspire and lose weight. They do make you perspire more. Your weight loss is water, not fat. When you eat or drink, you replace the water and weight.

Pills

Doctors will no longer prescribe pills to suppress appetite. They are dangerous. Pills do not change your eating habits.

Sauna baths

Some people like sauna baths because they help them to feel more relaxed. A good hot shower or bath can do the same thing. These baths can't take off fat or cure or prevent some diseases!

Body wraps

The body is wrapped in bandages soaked in a so-called 'magic solution'. It is claimed to make you lose 'inches' of fat. It won't.

As a teenager, Manuel Kimi was the school fatty. He weighed twice as much as the other boys, and ate three times as much. It wasn't until his twenties that he finally faced his problem—and when he went to his first Weight Watchers class, a special extension had to be added to the scales to weigh him! He was 223 kg (35 stone).

Following the Weight Watchers programme carefully, eating three sensible meals a day, Manuel began to lose weight steadily. At the same time he began exercising at the local gym. With the encouragement of the others in his class, he didn't have a single weight gain, or miss any meetings.

Manuel's determination grew as his goal of 77 kg (12 stone) approached. When he went home for Christmas his family couldn't believe their eyes, and he was interviewed on local radio. Finally his dream came true, and having lost 146 kg (23 stone), he was presented with a three-piece suit by Weight Watchers as a gift for a wonderful effort. Manuel regrets that he didn't do something about his weight during his teens. It is twice as hard for an adult to lose weight! His advice to any overweight teenager: 'Do something about it NOW!'

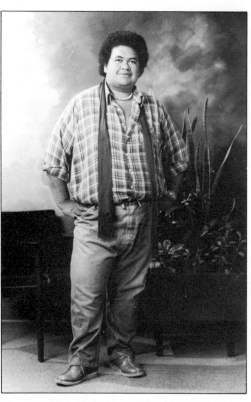

Manuel Kimi. When this photo was taken, he had already lost 38 kg (6 stone).

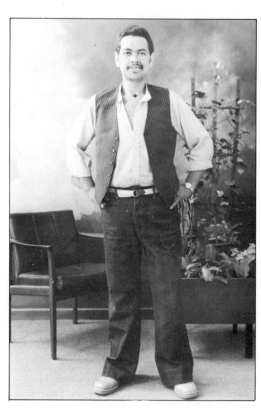

146 kg (23 stone) lighter!   *Photos of Manuel by courtesy of Weight Watchers*

As his story shows, even when Manuel was at his fattest he was able to begin an exercise programme. Some people try to lose weight just by cutting down on their food intake, but then they have to choose foods which only give them a few kilojoules. This means they end up eating a very narrow range of foods and find it very hard to keep going. Their food gets very boring. Remember the formula:

less food + more activity = weight goes down

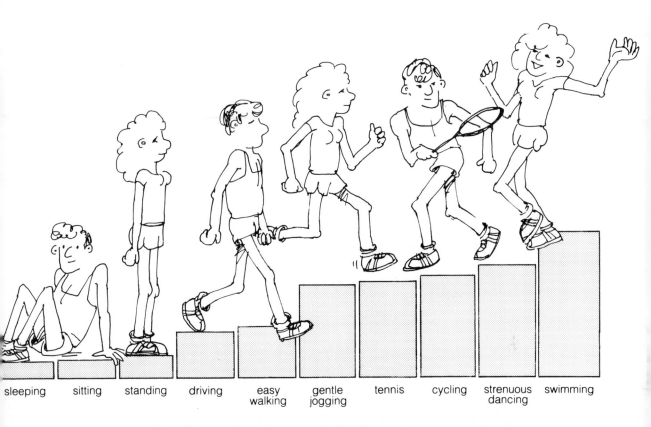

| sleeping | sitting | standing | driving | easy walking | gentle jogging | tennis | cycling | strenuous dancing | swimming |

How much energy different activities use up

You can't control your weight by diet alone. That is, not unless you're willing to eat very little food for the rest of your life.

You don't have to count kilojoules (Calories) to know what activities to do and which foods to eat. Find an activity you enjoy. It doesn't have to be running or swimming—it can be dancing or biking or walking or anything else energetic. Try to be active every day. At least three times a week is the minimum.

> Something active every day.
> Not enough unless you puff.

The diagram above shows how much energy different activities use up. The chart that follows shows you which foods you should choose to:
get in shape
stay slim
feel fine.

All you have to remember are the three colours of traffic lights—green, amber (yellow) and red. (This traffic light is upside down!)

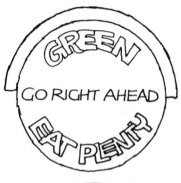

Fresh fruits, salads, vegetables including potatoes (not fried or roasted), whole grain cereals, bread (careful of the spread), fish and poultry (not fried), cottage cheese, skimmed or non-fat milk, plain yoghurt.

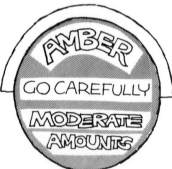

Meat, oily fish (like sardines), eggs, milk, cheese (there's more fat in cheese than in chocolate), rice, pasta with thick sauces, paté.

Foods high in fat*
Fried food, cheese, fat on meat, fish and chips, fat, butter, margarine, mayonnaise, crisps, nuts, pastries.
Foods high in Sugar
Sweets, chocolate, tinned fruit, jam, jelly, cooked puddings, cake, biscuits, soft drinks, alcohol.

---

*Fat and fatty foods give you the most kilojoules of all foods.

Check your favourite cheese for its fat content in the table below. Slimmers often make the mistake of filling up on cheese, not realising that most cheeses are very rich in fat.

Cheese	Fat Content (%)
Cottage cheese	4
Cheese spread	23
Edam type	23
Camembert type	23
Processed cheese	25
Danish Blue type	29
Cheddar type	34
Stilton type	40
Cream cheese	47

Here are some more fat-fighting hints to help you cut down on the energy value of the foods you eat. (You don't need to work out the kilojoule value of foods, but these 'specials' show you how easy it is to do.)

SPECIAL!

Don't reach for a biscuit every time you have a cup of tea or coffee. White coffee by itself gives you 80 kJ; coffee and a chocolate biscuit give you about 400 kJ. So you could . . .

SAVE 320 KJ

SPECIAL!

Icecream contains fat, so avoid it—you could substitute natural yoghurt on desserts. Four tinned apricot halves give you about 360 kJ; with icecream this goes up to 900 kJ. So you could . . .

SAVE 540 KJ

SPECIAL!

Stop frying most foods—grilling, casseroling, or poaching are better because they mean you eat less fat. Poached white fish is about 400 kJ per helping, compared with 1200 kJ fried. So you could . . .

SAVE 800 KJ

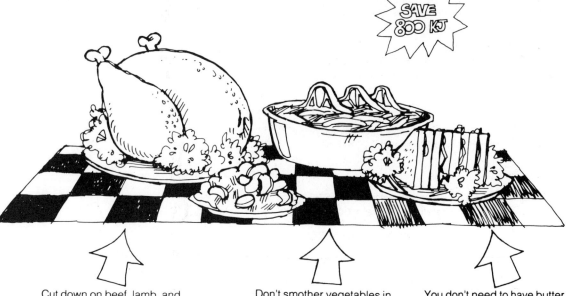

Cut down on beef, lamb, and pork. Choose chicken, fish, and shellfish more often—they contain much less fat.

Don't smother vegetables in butter when you serve them—try a sprinkling of lemon juice and fresh herbs instead.

You don't need to have butter and margarine in sandwiches—try it and see! If you're using a very dry filling, spread the bread, thinly with 'low-calorie' salad cream.

So you still want to go on a diet?

If you haven't yet reached your adult height and weight, check with your doctor or a dietitian before you go on any 'diet'.

Some 'diets' are dangerous for growing people.

Some diets you see in magazines are *harmful*. How do you know which diets are daft, dumb, damaging, or dangerous?

To protect yourself from fad* diets you need the 'handy' checklist below.

iets must be lived with. Avoid those containing only a few boring foods.

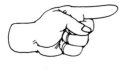
nclude these important foods? Fruit Cereals Bread Vegetables Potatoes

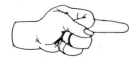
xercise must be part of any diet programme

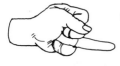
hree meals a day? (Or five or six smaller meals.)

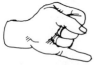
afety is most important. Be careful of any diet which promises quick weight loss or calls itself 'Dr Someone's Diet'.

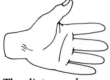
Nutritional Guidelines should be followed

The diet you choose should check out on all these points

*A fad diet is a *fashionable* diet or *craze*.

The diet you choose *must check out* on *all six* points.

ACTIVITIES

1   The table opposite gives details of some popular diets found in magazines, and published in books. In your exercise book, draw up a table like the one below. Check out each diet with your handy checklist. One has been done for you. Watch out for other diet plans, and check them over too.

Name/Description	Diet checklist points						Your Comments
	D	I	E	T	S	NG (Nutritional goals)	
1. 'Dr Atkins Diet Revolution'	×	×	×	✓	×	×	Unsafe Diet*
2. 'Bananas and Milk'							
3. 'F-Plan'							
4. Meal Replacements							
5. 'Weight Watchers'							
6. 'Grapefruit'							

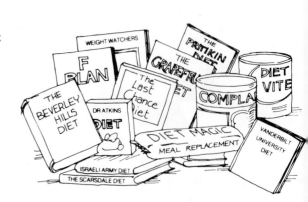

*In fact this diet is extremely dangerous. Because it gives you no carbohydrate, fibre, or natural sugar from fruit, it puts a big strain on body systems. Many medical people consider all high-protein and high-fat diets quite unsafe.

Diet	Suggested Menu
1 'Dr Atkins' High in animal foods like meat, eggs, cheese. These are mainly fat and protein. This diet bans fruit, cereals, vegetables (except for greens), and grains. No mention of exercise. Suggests you take extra vitamin pills. 'You can expect to lose 2–4 kg in the first week and 1–2 kg in the next weeks.'	*Breakfast* bacon eggs fried in butter cheese (50 g) tea or coffee, no milk *Lunch* small green salad oil and vinegar dressing hamburger (meat only) cheese (50 g) diet soda *Dinner* small green salad oil and vinegar dressing lamb chops courgettes (zucchini) cottage cheese coffee or tea, no milk
2 'Bananas and Milk' Eat bananas and milk as much as you like for 5 days.	Bananas and milk at every meal and for snacks.
3 'F-Plan' You *must* eat fibre filler, (3 sorts of bran and dried fruit mixed), and have 300 ml of non-fat milk and 2 pieces of fruit each day. Breakfast is the same each day. You set yourself a maximum kilojoule intake per day. You have a total intake of dietary fibre of 35–50 g per day. There is little choice.	*Breakfast* half the daily portion of fibre filler non-fat milk coffee or tea *Lunch* wholemeal sandwiches (2 slices bread; lettuce, meat, or fish) apple or orange *Dinner* 100 g lean meat large baked potato with yoghurt dressing green vegetable apple or orange Fibre filler as snack
4 'Meal Replacements' You make up drinks from a powder and have these drinks instead of usual meals. They contain fillers, vitamins, and mineral powders and are flavoured and coloured.	Replace at least one usual meal a day with the diet drink.

5   'Weight Watchers'

Dieters join a class of other dieters for a weekly fee.
The programme includes all the foods which may
be eaten. Encourages exercise ('Pep Step').
Changes eating habits.

Breakfast
orange juice
cereal, plain yoghurt
toast
coffee

Lunch
tunafish salad sandwich
milk
apple

Dinner
chicken
green beans, carrots
green salad
kiwi fruit
coffee or tea

6   'Grapefruit'

Grapefruit burns up fat! You eat half a grapefruit
before every meal.

Your normal meals—as long as you have half a
grapefruit before each meal.

2   Discuss these:
(a) If so many slimming diets promise successful
weight loss, why do new ones appear in
newspapers and magazines all the time?
(b) This is Darrell's training diet.

> 'Before the championships last weekend, I went on a diet so
> that I'd be lighter than him and in a different division. I was
> allowed oysters and steak, but I couldn't have any lollies. I
> missed having lollies.'

(c) Gary lost 57 of his 140 kilos in just over 9
months. Here's how he did it.

> 'I don't believe in faddy diets,' he says. He fasted for two
> weeks while he was in Asia, drinking only water. He came
> back, exercised a lot and now eats only one meal a day.
> Doesn't drink alcohol any more, spends time in a gym once
> a week, and jogs—he likes the high it gives although it
> 'bores me to tears'.

(d) Talk about what you have learnt from this
chapter, 'Eating Safely'. What surprised you most?
(e) Which diet is the best slimming diet?

3   *For you to do:*
(a) Find slimming diets from other people, or in
magazines, newspapers, and advertisements.
Paste them in your book. Using the checklist
evaluate them. Put any comments alongside.
(b) Work out a slimming diet. Describe the diet
and write down a menu for three days' meals.
Now check it against your handy checklist. How
does it compare? Six ticks? *Well done.*

6
'Have a drink'

Everything you drink, except water, soda water, and black coffee or tea, gives your body kilojoules. So nearly everything you drink counts as a kind of food. Now when most people think of 'drink' they think of alcohol. How does alcohol rate as a food? Alcohol gives the body kilojoules but *no other nutrients*. It is simply fattening.

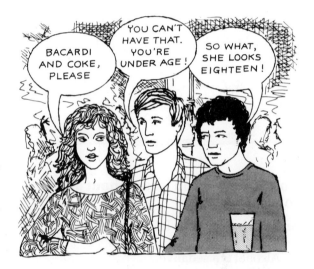

Average glass of alcohol	kJ	Food equivalent
beer 210 ml	420	1 doughnut
wine 90 ml	300	5 plain biscuits
spirits 20 ml (a single)	215	1 chocolate
spirits mixed with soft drink	588	12 potato crisps

Alcohol is more than just a drink. Alcohol matters to most adults.

Drinking alcohol is part of the way of life for most people, and for many of us it is one of life's pleasures. Some experts believe that moderate amounts (no more than two drinks a day) can benefit people's health. But many of us must be drinking more than this. There are an estimated 700,000 people in this country who are in trouble with their drinking. Those who are drinking a lot are harming themselves, and all the rest of us too. 75% of alcoholics have jobs and they cost industry around £2 billion a year in lost hours, accidents and hung-over work.

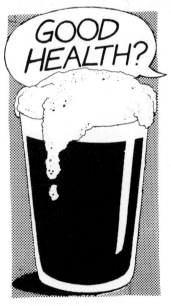

HOW LONG DOES IT TAKE TO RECOVER FROM JUST ONE DRINK?

WHAT PART DOES ALCOHOL PLAY IN THE DIET?

DOES ALCOHOL AFFECT YOUNG PEOPLE MORE THAN OLD?

WHAT'S THE SAFEST WAY TO DRINK?

HOW MUCH DRINKING CAN CAUSE SERIOUS DAMAGE?

How much do you know about alcohol and drinking?

Are these statements TRUE or FALSE?

1 Alcohol is a drug.
2 Alcohol is a sedative.
3 Alcohol is a stimulant (it peps you up).
4 Alcohol is fattening.
5 Most people in Britain drink alcohol.
6 Consumption of alcohol in this country continues to go up.
7 Alcohol mixed with fizzy drinks (such as tonic, cola, lemonade) acts faster in the body than alcohol mixed with water or juices.
8 The best cure for a hangover is another drink.
9 Alcohol has different effects on different people.
10 People get drunk from mixing drinks.
11 Alcohol improves driving skills.
12 Alcohol drunk during pregnancy will affect the unborn baby.

13 If you eat food while you are drinking, the alcohol is absorbed more quickly than on an empty stomach.
14 Drinking alcohol when you are cold increases your body temperature.
15 Alcohol abuse costs us all a lot of money each year.
16 You have to have at least five drinks before you get drunk.
17 You can sober up quickly if you have black coffee, or a cold shower.
18 You can die of alcohol poisoning.
19 You don't know any alcoholics.
20 Road accidents after drinking are the biggest cause of death in young men.

Here are the facts

1 TRUE. Alcohol is a drug which affects your brain and your body. It changes your behaviour. It is dangerous to mix alcohol with any other drug or medicine.

In a test with professional drivers, the more they had to drink the more certain they were that they could drive between moveable posts, and the less able they were to do it.

DAMN AND BLAST!

HE'S KNOCKED OVER HALF OF THEM!

2 TRUE. Because alcohol is chemically a close relation to ether it is very like an anaesthetic. It acts as a depressant on the brain, and it slows you down.

3 FALSE. See above. It feels as though you are pepped up but this is because your perception is changed.

4 TRUE. Alcohol adds kilojoules but has no other nutrients. If you drink alcohol regularly and eat your usual food you will put on weight.

5 TRUE. Only about 15 per cent never drink.

6 TRUE.

7 TRUE.

8 FALSE. There is no cure for a hangover.

9 TRUE. Young people are more quickly affected. They show aggressive or stupid behaviour sooner.

10 FALSE. The amount of alcohol you drink is what decides how drunk you get.

11 FALSE. People often think they are driving better. But tests show differently! The drunker drivers are, the less they realise how incapable they are. Alcohol increases your confidence because it decreases your judgement and sense of responsibility.

12 TRUE. Babies whose mothers drink heavily during pregnancy can be harmed mentally and physically. When a pregnant woman drinks, the baby has a drink as well! Alcohol passes straight from her body into the developing baby. The more she drinks, the greater chance there is of damage to the baby.

13 FALSE. Food is very important! Food slows down the rate at which alcohol is absorbed into the body.

14 FALSE. Not only false but dangerous! When people suffer from extreme cold, exposure, or hypothermia the body tries to protect itself by closing off the blood vessels in the limbs. This keeps the blood in the 'core' of the body. Alcohol relaxes the blood vessels in the limbs and lets the blood flow back from the warm core. Then the body temperature drops even lower.

15 TRUE. Every taxpayer pays—for the cost of treatment facilities for alcoholics, hospitals

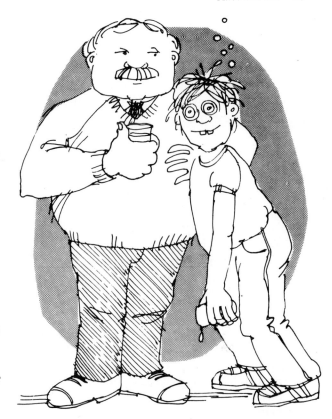

for the victims of alcohol-related accidents, and for prisons for those who commit serious crimes after drinking.

16 FALSE. Even one drink can make you drunk. It depends on your age, size, personality, and previous experience with alcohol.

17 FALSE. Black coffee, cold showers, and fresh air are often used to try and sober people up. The only effects these have is to produce a wide-awake cold drunk. There is no way to speed up the rate at which your body gets rid of alcohol.

18 TRUE. People who drink large amounts of alcohol in a short time can die of alcohol poisoning.

19 FALSE. At least one person in fifty is an alcoholic. Alcoholics can be difficult to spot because they can drink large quantities of alcohol without showing the usual signs of being drunk.

20 TRUE!

Score box—how did YOU score?

15–20   You have enough knowledge to protect yourself and make responsible decisions about alcohol.

10–15   Room for improvement.

5–10   You need to know more facts about alcohol. You believe too many myths.

0–5   Your lack of knowledge could be hurting other people, and yourself. Find out the facts, today!

Research has shown that workers who have drunk between 1 and 3 pints of beer have considerably more accidents.

Coping with alcohol

Alcohol is a very powerful drug. These people have to be especially careful about its effects on their bodies:
    females
    small-framed people
    infrequent drinkers
    overweight people
    emotional people
    people physically sensitive to alcohol.
    As you can see in the diagram, alcohol affects your brain and other parts of your body too. You feel on top of the world, and even in control of yourself. But other people might not think that you are the life and soul of the party.

Everybody may like a drink.
But nobody likes a drunk.

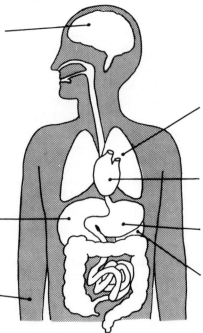

Your **brain** is slowed down. This changes the way your senses of touch, taste, sight, smell, and hearing work. It alters your emotions and upsets your ability to make judgements. Messages to your muscles travel more slowly and you may stagger, stumble, stutter, or slur your words. The brain cells are often affected by drinking large amounts of alcohol.

The **liver** removes most of the alcohol from your blood. It removes about a glassful an hour. Too much alcohol will damage it, causing scarring (cirrhosis).

Sweat glands all over your body help to get rid of alcohol as your perspire.

Your **lungs** help to get rid of alcohol as you breathe out. This is why a breathalyser can show how much you have drunk.

Alcohol in your blood is pumped all over your body by the **heart.**

Your **stomach** may be irritated and upset by alcohol. You may feel sick, and vomit.

The **pancreas** is damaged by too much alcohol. This can cause diabetes.

How your body copes with alcohol

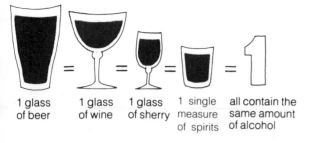

1 glass of beer	1 glass of wine	1 glass of sherry	1 single measure of spirits	all contain the same amount of alcohol

In the cartoon Greg is feeling great. But next morning he will wake up feeling awful. He will have a hangover. His body will try to get rid of the alcohol he drank last night.

People often feel ashamed of how they acted while they were drinking. Anyone who can't remember what he or she did for all or part of that time has had a blackout. Blackouts mean brain damage. See page 70.

An average glass of one one sort of liquor contains about the same amount of alcohol as an average glass of other sorts of liquor (the glass makers design them that way). Note that spirits are drinks such as gin, whisky, brandy, bourbon, rum, and tequila

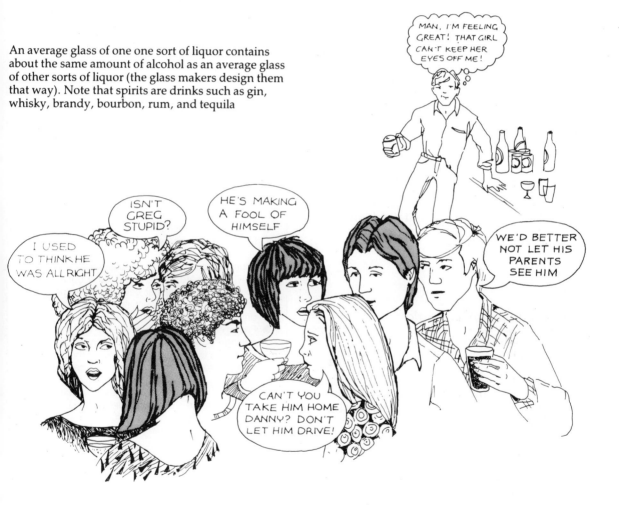

To Drink or not to Drink

Often you'll be in situations where people expect you to drink. This doesn't mean you have to drink a lot, or anything at all. It means you have a choice! It's *your* choice.

If you choose to drink . . .

1   Understand alcohol

People who drink alcohol responsibily drink slowly, limit the amount, and never lose control of their behaviour. They don't drink alone.

2   Obey the laws concerning drinking

With a few exceptions alcohol cannot be sold to people under 18.

3   Face the risk of drinking too much

The possibilities include drunkenness, embarrassment, blackouts, hangovers, motor accidents, and even unwanted pregnancy.

4   Respect non-drinkers

They made a choice too.

If you choose not to drink . . .

1   Know your reason

Drinking may be against the rules or customs of your family, school, or religion. You may choose not to drink because you do not like the taste, or the effects. You may have other good reasons.

2   Don't apologise for saying 'no thanks' to a drink

Say it calmly, casually, and firmly. Like this: 'No thanks, a soft drink for me, please', or 'Make mine orange, please'. There is no need to explain or make excuses.

3   Expect others to respect your choice

Your choice should be respected just as you respect theirs.

The Happy Drinking Code

Most of us learn about drinking from watching other people, and sometimes learning from our own mistakes. Usually if we have too much to drink we laugh it off. We seldom try to work out why, this particular time, we 'overdid it'.

Advertisements suggest that we may be sexier or more sophisticated or feel more relaxed if we drink certain types of alcohol. No one is sexy or sophisticated when they are drunk or have a hangover, so here are some points to remember if you use alcohol to add relaxation to your social life.

- Don't drink when you're going to drive or use machinery.
- Choose coffee, tea or non-alcoholic drinks instead of alcohol sometimes.
- If you drink with people who regularly buy rounds for each other, it's easy to end up drinking more than you want. You could say you'd rather just get your own. Others in the group may prefer that too, because buying rounds can get very expensive. Alternatively, drink slowly so that your glass stays fuller longer. 'I'm OK this time,' you can say. Choose small measures like half pints rather than pints, or alternate between alcoholic and non-alcoholic drinks.
- Try setting yourself limits for particular occasions. Decide how much you really want to drink before you start. Then stick to that limit. You can keep count of your drinks in various ways: write them down on a card, make marks on a beermat with your thumbnail, transfer coins from one pocket to another. Don't lose count and you won't end up drinking more than you want.
- Pace your drinking throughout the evening. If you manage to keep to your limits, give yourself a reward - a visit to the cinema, new clothes, an extra hour in bed on Sunday morning - something you'd not usually allow yourself.
- If you feel you're likely to drink more than you really want to, create a deliberate delay. Go somewhere for five minutes. Say to yourself, 'I'm in control of my own life.' You are. Often you'll be better able to stick to your plan.
- Remember that getting drunk doesn't make you tall, rich, strong, handsome, smart, witty, sophisticated or sexy.

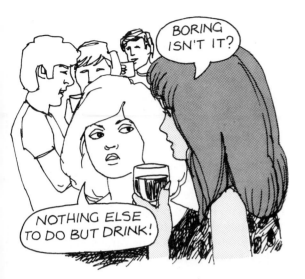

Heavy drinking isn't a sign of a successful party

Host's Code

Parties are for fun. If you are the host you need to provide more than just drink.

- Serve plenty of food—not just at supper time. It's a good idea to have food out all the time so people can help themselves.
- Provide music and entertainment for your guests.
- Have plenty of non-alcoholic drinks for people who want to take it easy. Soft drinks, juices and fruit punch are popular with everyone. There are recipes for party drinks at the end of this chapter.
- Let people help themselves to drink.

It's NOT FRIENDLY to
Insist that guests drink
Top up glasses
Be heavy-handed.

It's FRIENDLY to
Serve snacks and coffee before people leave
Stop anyone driving if you think he/she has had too much. Call a taxi or ask a sober guest to drive, or offer a bed for the night. You may save your friend's life.

Most young people think they are too young to be alcoholic. They may have seen parents drinking over a number of years without becoming alcoholic. It's difficult for them to believe that they have a problem but even people in their early teens can be alcoholics.

Questions about alcoholism

Q: What is alcoholism? What causes it?
Worried Grandson

A: Alcoholism is a disease. Sufferers can't control the amount they drink, even though it may be hurting them. The damage may be to their bodies, their minds, their relationships with other people, to their work, and to their security.

Apart from the fact that it is caused by drinking lots of alcohol, no one really knows why someone *becomes* an alcoholic. Doctors now think that it may run in families, though this is only part of the story.

Q: How can you tell if you might be an alcoholic? What are the signs?
Mike S.

A: Not everyone develops alcoholism quickly. For some people it is a long, slow process. Many recovering and recovered alcoholics say that they now know that their drinking was never normal, right from the first time they had anything to drink. The important thing is to know the signs of problem drinking, and to get help if there *is* a problem.

There are several early signs of problem drinking which may mean alcoholism. The important thing to remember is that alcoholics do not necessarily drink during the day, on the job, before breakfast, or even every day. But when they do drink, problem drinkers:

- Drink FASTER than others
- Don't stop after ONE drink
- May GULP drinks rather than sip
- Work out ways of getting EXTRA drinks when drinking with others

- SPEND quite a lot on alcohol
- Are not TRUTHFUL about the quantity they drink
- May be GUILTY about drinking behaviour
- Make PROMISES about drinking less
- DEPEND on drinks, especially at a certain time
- Have BLACKOUTS (cannot remember things that happen during drinking).

Q: Where would I get help for someone with a terrible drinking problem?

Rebecca

A: If you, your friend, or someone in your family needs help with a drinking problem, your first approach could be to go to:
- Your youth club leader or a teacher you know well
- An adult you can trust
- Your church minister/elder
- Samaritans
- A local teenage advice telephone line
- A Doctor.

These people will refer you to the best help available for your problem.
- For access to a national network of over 40 local council and advice centres:
  National Council on Alcoholism,
  3 Grosvenor Crescent, London SW1
    Tel: (01) 235 4182
- For the family and friends of problem drinkers:
  Al Anon Family Groups, 61 Great Dover Street, London SE1 4YF
    Tel: (01) 403 0888
- For help if you've got a drinking problem:
  Alcoholics Anonymous, PO Box 514,
  11 Redcliffe Gardens, London SW10 9BQ
    Tel: (01) 352 9779

  In Ireland 152 Lisburn Road, Belfast BT9 6AJ
    Tel: Belfast (0232) 681084

  In Wales Tel: Cardiff (0222) 373939
- For advice, information and counselling:
  The Accept Clinic, 200 Seagrave Road, London SW6
    Tel: (01) 381 3155

There is also a group called 'Alateen' which

offers support to teenagers who have an alcoholic parent. The Salvation Army tries to care for some of those whose lives have been wrecked by their addiction to alcohol.

Q: I have heard that alcohol can damage your brain. Is this so? How much is dangerous? What does it do?

Sandra

A: Too much alcohol, too often, damages the brain. It inflames the brain cells and, tough as they are, the cells can in time die. There is no known reprieve! You can't tell how much damage has already happened to your own brain cells—the only symptoms will be **blackouts**. If you forget what's happened during drinking, that's a blackout. You may be unable to remember recent events, or have blanks in your memory—these are all signs of too much alcohol.

Not just the brain, but the whole nervous system is disturbed by alcohol. Heavy drinkers may become confused, have convulsions, the 'DTs', delusions, and hallucinations. If the brain has been badly damaged the person becomes a helpless invalid, who can never recover.

The stomach, liver, pancreas, and other body organs are also damaged by too much alcohol, but that's another story.

ACTIVITIES

1   Design a badge or T-shirt slogan that will help people to understand about alcohol.

2   What's a 'beer pot'? Why do *men* get 'beer pots'? What do women get?

3   Christchurch secondary school students were shown a 'Road Show' performance about the effects of drinking and driving. Afterwards, some of the girls made a blacklist. On the blacklist were the names of boys that the girls wouldn't drive with. Why? What do you think of this?

4   (a) Many alcohol companies and outlets sponsor events. They put up money and usually have big advertising signs at the events they sponsor. What could be the effects of this advertising?

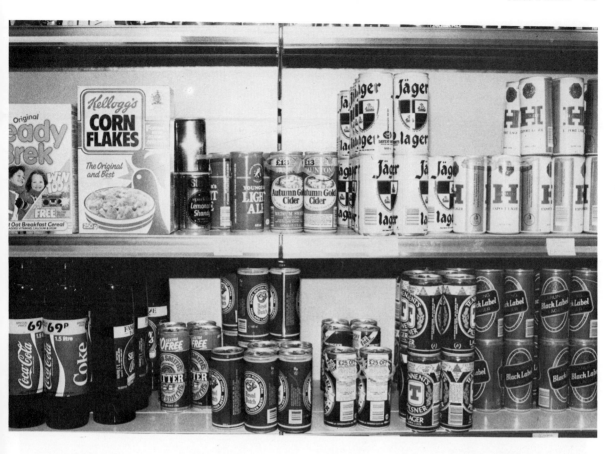

(b) Read what these 15 year old pupils had to say about alcohol. Talk about these experiences.

James: 'We had a bit from each bottle so that they couldn't tell what we had done when they got back.'
Susan: 'I didn't know what to ask for when they said "What do you want to drink?"'
Catherine: 'They used to take me into the pub with them even though I was under age.'
Nick: 'He was sick on the bus on the way home.'

(c) Collect alcohol advertisements which give you the impression that you will be sexy, sophisticated, witty, lovable, interesting, attractive, popular, or better in some way, if you drink a particular brand. What age groups are the ads aimed at? Design some advertisements that tell the truth about drinking.
(d) Discuss or debate the proposal 'that alcohol advertising should be banned'.
(e) Should alcohol be sold in supermarkets?

5 Some ways that have been used to promote moderate drinking are shown below.
(a) The advertisement on page 72 is promoted by an association of liquor companies. What are the messages? Do you think it is manly to drink?
(b) A brewery has developed family restaurants open 7 days a week, 7.30 a.m. to 10 p.m. The restaurant sells meals and alcohol. There are bars where people wait for seats in the restaurant. Would this encourage moderate drinking?

6 *Role Play*
The host at the party is trying to make the guests drink a lot.
● One guest doesn't want to drink at all.
● Another guest wants to drink sensibly.
● Yet another has had too much and wants to drive home.

7 What's it like to *hit bottom*? Contact your nearest group of Alcoholics Anonymous and ask if a member can come and talk to the class.

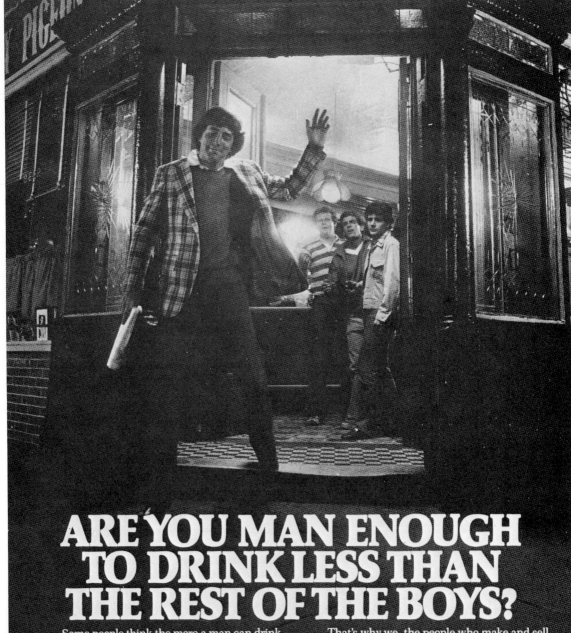

ARE YOU MAN ENOUGH TO DRINK LESS THAN THE REST OF THE BOYS?

Some people think the more a man can drink, the more of a man he is. However, it usually works the other way around.

Men who drink to build up their egos, end up putting themselves down.

The guy who claims he can drink everyone under the table looks pretty low. Especially if he gets there.

The hero who thinks it's macho to drink like a fish is regarded by sensible people as an animal.

That's why we, the people who make and sell distilled spirits, urge you to use our products with common sense. If you choose to drink, drink responsibly.

A real man has the strength to say no when he's had enough.

Distilled Spirits Council of the U.S. (DISCUS), 1300 Pennsylvania Building, Washington, D.C. 20004

IT'S PEOPLE WHO GIVE DRINKING A BAD NAME.

Courtesy Distilled Spirits Council of the U.S.

8 There are some people who are regularly arrested by the police for being 'drunk and disorderly'. Is the treatment they receive suitable and adequate?

9 What would *you* do? You are the Minister in Charge of Alcohol. The Cabinet has told you to reduce the cost of alcohol to the country—in lives lost in accidents on the roads, by drowning, and in industry; in hospital costs in caring for those damaged by alcohol; in prisons. What actions will you take?

Party Drinks

Pineapple Punch

300 ml left-over tea, strained
150 ml lemon juice
450 ml orange juice (squeezed, canned, or cartoned)
2 tablespoons lime cordial
250 g sugar
450 ml pineapple juice
2.5 l ginger ale (2 × 1.25 l bottles)
several sprigs mint

1. Crush mint in a big vessel—plastic or stainless steel
2. Add warm, strained tea. Cool.
3. Add fruit juices.
4. Add ginger ale before serving.

Ginger Tingle

1 tablespoon sugar
2 glasses water
2 glasses grapefruit juice (cartoned or canned)
1 × 1.25 l bottle ginger ale

1. Boil sugar and water 5 minutes, cool.
2. Add fruit juice. Chill.
3. Add ginger ale before serving.

High Flyer

1 tablespoon honey
1 orange thinly sliced
1 large carton grapefruit juice
mint sprigs
500 ml boiling water
soda water

1. Put mint sprigs in a bowl. Add honey, orange slices, and boiling water.
2. Cool. Add grapefruit juice.
3. Serve on ice in tall glasses. Top with soda water.

Bloody Shame

Mix chilled tomato juice with a dash of worcester sauce, salt, pepper, and a squeeze of lemon juice. Sprinkle with celery salt.

7
Keep moving!

If someone offered you something which could
> make you look great and feel better
> give you confidence in yourself
> help you lose weight
> build up your muscles
> give you a great night's sleep
> help you give up smoking
> help you relax
> give you more energy
> help you have more fun
> give you a natural high

and was very cheap, would you take it?

Of course you would.

There *is* something that can do all these things. It is readily available, and is practically free to anyone who will choose to make the effort. It is *simple physical exercise.*

What exercise can't do for you:

- It can't take off weight (unless you reduce your food intake too)
- It can't take away your problems, although it will help you to handle them better
- It can't change your personality, though it can help you change your shape
- It can't make you popular, but it can help you meet people.

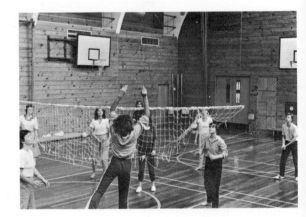

When you were little you used up a lot of energy and kept fit by just playing. Young children use the big muscles of their bodies in their free play.

Primary school children still play a lot of games but they start to do team sports and join clubs too—like gym, pony clubs, soccer teams, and ballet. Children of this age can control their movements better. By the time people are at secondary school they get organised sport and P.E. as part of the curriculum, and can get into sports teams. Their control of their muscle movement is now well developed.

When people leave school they may not be able to take part in organised activities. They need to find activities they can do in their own time which are satisfying and fun. Use

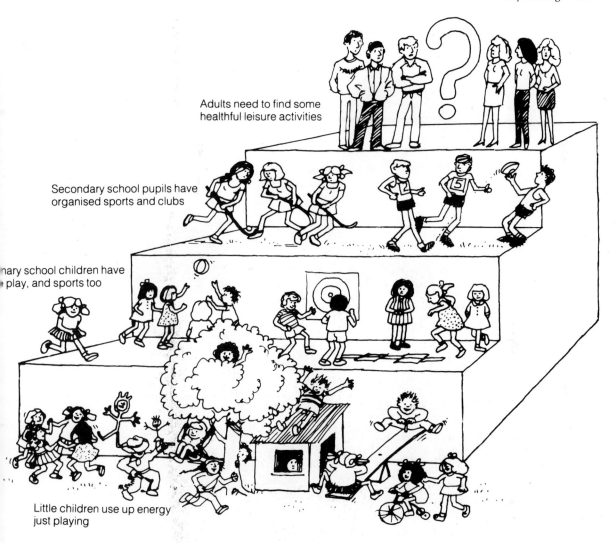

Adults need to find some healthful leisure activities

Secondary school pupils have organised sports and clubs

...nary school children have
... play, and sports too

Little children use up energy
just playing

the chance you have at school to try out as many activities as you can. There may be trips or visits to different activities or clubs in your area. Students from many schools have been white-water canoeing, yachting, skiing, skating, climbing, and gliding.

Your body deserves the best care you can give it! It must get enough physical activity. Even if you've not found any particular sport that suits you yet, you need to find some way of keeping fit.

Maybe you feel fit, and are pretty active. Fine! Your body was designed to be like this. You will want to make sure you keep it that way for the rest of your life. Many people who were fit when they were at school playing organised or team sports find it hard to keep them up.

- Ian found that his job stopped him playing competition hockey. He had to travel out of town.
- Grace gave up netball at top team level because it took up too much time. She wanted to spend time on her other interests.
- Steve gave up rugby because his achilles tendon injury wouldn't heal.
- Sarah gave up competition swimming when a younger girl got her place in the team.

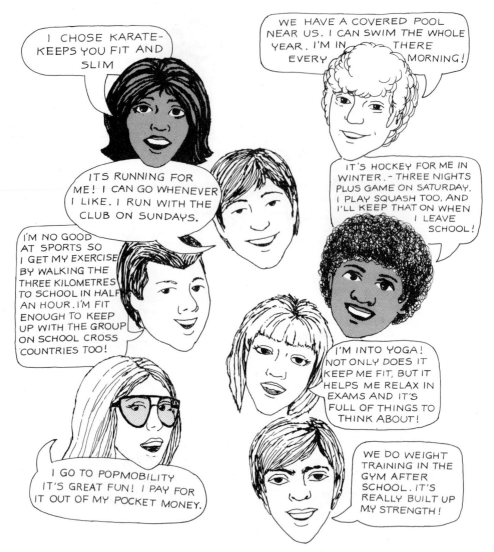

Skating, rowing, tennis, jogging, netball, dance, judo, football, gymnastics, softball, surfing—it's up to you

The best exercise for you is
    The one you enjoy most
    The one you can keep on with for many years
    One you can do flat-out for half an hour three times a week (standing in goal three times a week won't help your fitness much)
    One that raises your pulse rate.

Starting an exercise programme?

Build up gradually. If you do too much on the first day you will get stiff and sore muscles. You could even give up the programme! Always do warm-up exercises. Ask your P.E. teacher or send for the Health Education Council leaflet 'Look after Yourself'.

An exercise programme can build muscles.

Neil was very thin. He felt embarrassed. He began to do weight training at the gym. At home he filled large empty detergent bottles with water and used them for his training.
Neil went on a body-building eating programme too*. He has started to fill out and he feels much happier with himself. He is more confident.

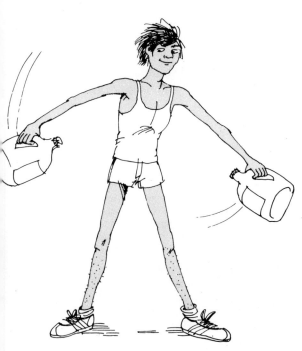

Exercise can help relieve menstrual cramps. Active women have less trouble with periods.

Hazel is in a school netball team, and gets plenty of exercise. Even so she sometimes finds it painful when her period starts. Her mother used to make her sit with a hot-water bottle. But her P.E. teacher suggested some exercise would be better. It worked! The sitting had made the pain worse.
Exercise in the fresh air can take away headaches—it is better than taking headache pills.

Chris often got headaches at school, especially around exam time. Chris found, quite by accident, that walking home cured the headaches.

Exercise can help you lose weight by using up more energy, and by suppressing your appetite.

Dawn had tried every 'diet' in the book. She could never stick to them. Since she started swimming every day she has found that she doesn't feel hungry. Her weight is now right for her height.

Exercise can help you give up smoking. Smoking and exercise don't mix! The more you enjoy exercise the less you'll want to smoke.

Scott gave up smoking after he began training for a local fun run. He found that he needed all the breath he could get! Scott felt so good after each run that he didn't want anything to spoil the 'high' feeling he got. His performance is improving.

Exercise can help you to relax and sleep better.

Tim's mother nagged him. Tim used to yell back and get really angry! One day he stormed out of the house and went for a run. He soon felt better. He could cope with Mum and he slept better too. Now Tim runs regularly. It helps him relax, and get rid of tension.

Exercise helps you get more fun.

- Paul made new friends at orienteering. He was shy but he found it easy to talk with the others about map-reading and the course.
- After a dance troupe gave a performance at school Craig, Gina, and Joe decided to join a modern dance group. They really enjoyed it.
- Robert tried out his cousin's windsurfer. It was fun! Robert was so excited he started building one himself, and met a whole lot of new friends.

*See Body Builder's Bonus, p 46, Chapter 4.

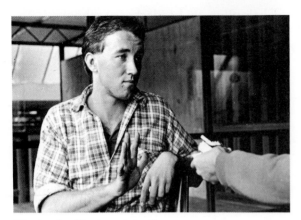

'No thanks, I'm in training!'

Exercise gives you more energy. People often think that exercise makes you tired, but only unfit people who try to do too much all at once get tired. If you are fit you will find that you can do more and that you have more energy.

- Ramon used to be so tired when he got home that all he did was look at TV. He started riding with his friends. His new fitness makes him feel less tired and ready for anything.
- Zoe got a new puppy. The puppy had to be exercised every day. Zoe was surprised to find that she enjoyed the time out. She felt better, and got so much energy that she (and the puppy) started jogging.

REGULAR EXERCISE IS THE KEY TO FITNESS

Enjoy yourself

Choose a form of exercise that you enjoy, so that the activity will be a pleasure and not a chore.

Be active

Use the stairs instead of the lift. Park a few blocks away from your destination; it may be quicker and more enjoyable to walk than to waste time hunting for a close parking space. Take every opportunity to be active.

Stretch

When you have been sitting or standing for a while stretch, relax, take a deep breath and relax again. Your body will enjoy the movement and you will feel refreshed.

Be supple

Take up an exercise that increases your flexibility (e.g. swimming, judo). Do these exercises every other day, or more often if you feel like it. You will soon notice that your muscles and joints are working better and your overall co-ordination has improved.

Be fit

Have an energetic workout three or four times a week (e.g. brisk walking, cycling, jogging, swimming)—the sort of exercise that raises your pulse rate and makes you breathe deeply.

Be sensible

Choose a form of exercise that is appropriate to your age and ability. Do some warming-up exercises first then start out slowly and work up to a reasonably energetic level. Don't overdo things and injure yourself.

The expense is up to you

Your exercise costs can be as simple or as expensive as your budget and inclination allow. The range goes from the price of a skipping rope, through the basic equipment for your favourite sport.

Keep it up

To make a worthwhile contribution to your health your exercise must be kept up regularly (three times a week or more).

Rethink your priorities

Don't make excuses about being about being too busy to exercise. Your own health is every bit as important as your other commitments. Rearrange your day, make time to exercise.

Make regular activity part of your life

Take up an active hobby or sport—fishing, tramping, gardening, orienteering, etc.—enjoy it with your family and friends.

from a booklet, 'Enjoying Life'*

*Published by The National Heart Foundation of New Zealand, The New Zealand Council for Recreation and Sport, and The Chemists' Guild of New Zealand Inc.

ACTIVITIES

1 You want to get the benefits from exercise. How can you decide which is the best activity for you? Check off your attitude towards different activities by completing this checklist in your exercise book. There are no right or wrong answers.

In your exercise book, rule up the table below.

	Rating		
Question	A	B	C
1 Social	☐	☐	☐
2 Enjoyment	☐	☐	☐
3 Training	☐	☐	☐
4 Competition	☐	☐	☐
5 Health	☐	☐	☐
6 Appearance	☐	☐	☐
7 Relaxation	☐	☐	☐

Answer the following questions. Put a tick in the correct box for each 'Yes'.

1 Do you:
A enjoy activities done in large groups?
B dislike activities you have to do by yourself?
C like sports and exercises you can do with two or three others?

2 Do you:
A enjoy activities that are exciting?
B dislike serious competition?
C think most activities are fun?

3 Do you:
A enjoy exercises that make you work hard?
B like activities that force you to do your best?
C dislike exercise and sports that are too easy?

4 Do you:
A like to compete?
B like activities that compare you with others?
C like winning?

5 Do you:
A enjoy activities that help you get healthy?
B enjoy activities that help you get physically fit?
C dislike staying in one place during the activity?

6 Do you:
A enjoy activities that are good for your build or your figure?
B want to improve the way you look?
C avoid activities that won't help you improve your appearance?

7 Do you:
A enjoy activities that help you relax?
B dislike activities that make you feel nervous?
C enjoy sports and games which make you feel at ease?

Now assess the sorts of activities for you. Remember this is an individual assessment. There are no right and wrong answers.

1 Three ticks means you enjoy exercise and games involving others. Pick at least one team sport. No ticks or just one tick? Then individual activities are for you.

2 People with two or three ticks here play sport for fun.

3 People with three ticks like to see what they can do physically. Take up some serious training.

4 People with three ticks here like to see how they compare with other people. Some sports are very competitive. If you got no (or one) tick here, avoid competitive activities.

5 Three ticks—or even two—mean you exercise for health and fitness, and for feeling good.

6 Three ticks here means you believe exercise will make you look better.

7 Three ticks—you need exercise to reduce stress and help you relax.

2 What other things do you have to think about in choosing a suitable and enjoyable activity? Discuss this statement by Professor Don Beaven: 'In Scandinavian countries and North America a lean body image is not only healthier, but is a mark of national self-pride and self-determination.'

What did the Professor mean? How could we develop pride in our physical image?

3 Arrange for the class to survey all the indoor and outdoor recreational and sports facilities (clubs, parks, gyms, etc.) within a 20 minute walk or bus, train, or bike ride from your school.
(a) Find out what it costs to use each facility. Who owns it? Who can use it?
(b) Find out the approximate age of the **oldest** participant. What age are **most** of the people who do the activity? Do they encourage school students to join them?

(c) In your exercise book make an alphabetical list of the activities you found. Rate each one on the following features:

Is it for individuals or teams?
Is it competitive or not?
Is it all-weather or seasonal?
Does it cost a lot to join?
Is it cheap or free?
How much equipment do you need? How much does it cost? Can it be hired?

(d) Circle any activity you would like to try now or when you leave school.

(e) If you can arrange it, try out at least *one* new activity.

4   Look in your local newspaper. Find advertisements for clubs and sports fixtures, and reports of sporting events. Can you find any more activities to add to your survey? Rate them in the same way.

5   Invite people to talk about their club activities. Ask if small groups can try out the activity. Can you arrange a weekend trip? Add any other sports or activities you have discovered to your alphabetical list. Rate them in the same way.

6   *For You to Do*

If you did the survey using your home as the base, not your school, could you include more activities?

Put yourself in the picture! Draw a step diagram like the one on page 75 in this chapter to show the active things you did when you were at primary school. On the next step show the active things including sports and recreation activities that you do now. On the top step list some active things you could do when you leave school.

8
'What's your poison?'

You know that eating a variety of food, a good exercise programme, keeping safe, and looking after yourself can help you feel fine. You choose to do these things. But sometimes your sensible lifestyle can be spoiled. It can be poisoned by drugs.

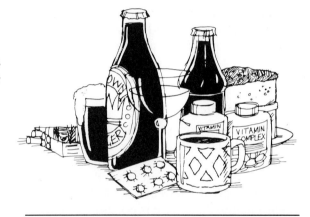

What is a drug?

Marijuana? Heroin? Cocaine? LSD? Other illegal substances? You might think of these, when you think of drugs. Aspirin? Cough mixture? Laxatives? Vitamin pills? These are drugs you can get from a chemist. Tobacco? Alcohol? Coca Cola? Tea? Coffee? Lots of things we take or use every day are drugs, too.

A drug is a substance that, when put into your body, can change the way your body works.

- Medicines are drugs.
- Coffee, tea, and colas all contain a stimulant called caffeine. But there is nothing illegal about drinking a cup of coffee or drinking a bottle of cola!
- Alcohol and tobacco are drugs. These two drugs are non-medical drugs, legal for adults (but not for children and teenagers).
- Illegal drugs include heroin, cocaine, marijuana, and LSD. They change your feelings and behaviour, your perceptions, and even your body's chemistry.

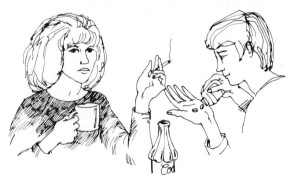

There are four drugs being taken by the people in this picture. What are they? They are not the sort of things most people think of when anyone mentions drugs

Medicines are drugs

Your healthy body usually heals itself. It can cure infections, mend broken bones, and heal diseases. It uses food, sleep, and relaxation, as well as its built-in defences, to do this.

Sometimes your body needs help to make you better. This is when drugs are used. You can buy some drugs from the chemist, such as cough mixture, aspirins, and travel sickness pills. They can be used to treat and prevent minor illnesses and infections. But if you don't get better after a few days, go to the doctor.

The doctor may give you a prescription. You have to take the prescription to the chemist where a qualified pharmacist will make it up. Some drugs are very strong and could cause a lot of damage if you took the wrong dose, or used it too often, or too little.

Too much medicine

Too much laxative can irritate the bowel. (You won't need a laxative at all if you have enough fibre in your diet.) Too much aspirin (or other pain reliever) can cause the stomach to bleed. It can also damage the kidneys. Too much Vitamin A, D, or E is poisonous. These vitamins are stored in the body.*

Too little

Some drugs take time to act. Antibiotics, such as penicillin, can make you feel better so quickly that you forget that the whole course is needed to kill all the disease-causing bacteria and clear up your infection.

Too strong

Certain drugs are powerful. Some can affect your blood, some can cause an allergic reaction, others can make you feel sick or dizzy. This is why many drugs can only be prescribed by your doctor who knows you and your medical history.

When you pick up your made-up prescription it will have a label with your

*If you think you need vitamins, ask your doctor. Never take them without medical advice.

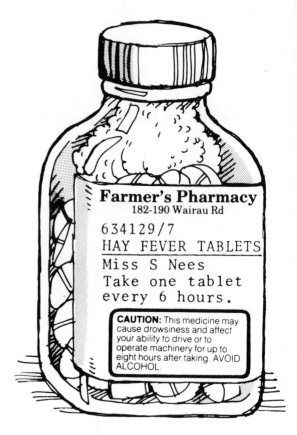

Farmer's Pharmacy
182-190 Wairau Rd
634129/7
HAY FEVER TABLETS
Miss S Nees
Take one tablet
every 6 hours.

CAUTION: This medicine may cause drowsiness and affect your ability to drive or to operate machinery for up to eight hours after taking. AVOID ALCOHOL.

Many of the drugs prescribed for allergies, hay fever, car sickness, sinus problems, and colds carry warnings

name, the name and amount of the drug, and how to take it. There may be an extra label which tells how to store the drug, or to warn you against doing certain things while you are taking it.

Many drugs **interact** with others in unexpected ways. They may speed up or have a stronger effect than on their own.

Sandra Nees likes a glass of wine or beer sometimes. But when she gets hay fever she drinks fruit juice instead. Why?

Any drugs taken by a pregnant woman, especially in the first three months of pregnancy, can affect an unborn child. Even the tablets or medicine she took when she was not pregnant can damage the baby. Doctors nowadays advise mothers-to-be to avoid alcohol, cigarettes, and even limit the coffee they drink.

Herbal remedies

Before there was modern medicine people relied a lot on herbal medicines to give them relief. Some herbal medicines are useless, while others may give some relief from minor complaints. They contain the ingredients of certain modern drugs in raw form. Some people may feel better because they believe the medicine will do them good!

It is against the law to claim that any product can cure certain diseases such as arthritis, cancer, heart disease, tuberculosis, poliomyelitis, or pneumonia. Some sellers of herbal medicines don't exactly break the law but they certainly bend it a bit! The labels on the bottles or packet themselves don't make any claims to cure. But the sellers put charts or leaflets on the shelves beside the medicines claiming that the product will cure or prevent different diseases. Sometimes the shop assistants will make the claims to the customers too.

Taking your medicine

Follow the Sensible Medicine Code:
- Always read the directions carefully and take the exact dose. The doctor prescribes the amount and kind of drug to suit the age and weight of the patient
- If your doctor has prescribed medicine for you, finish the course—even if you do feel better. If in doubt, ask your doctor or chemist
- Tell your doctor or chemist of any side-effects you have noticed
- Take your own medicine! It was specially prescribed to deal with *your* illness. Don't offer it to a friend—and don't 'borrow' his or hers
- If you're advised not to drink, drive, or operate machinery while taking a medicine—don't. It's dangerous
- Don't keep unused prescribed medicines or over-the-counter medicines with an expiry date that has expired. Return them to the chemist or throw them down the toilet—not into the rubbish bin or on the fire

- Keep all medicines, including aspirin, locked away from children. Use child-proof containers too
- Never let a child get hold of medicines. To children, brightly coloured tablets are just like sweets.

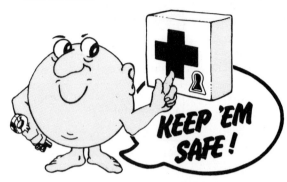

What if the medicine doesn't work?

If you haven't got better, ask yourself—did you
- take the medicine exactly as it was prescribed?
- tell the doctor the *real* problem? (For example, people can have bad headaches when really they feel stressed.)

You did? Go back to the doctor and explain how you feel. Sometimes just talking to someone can help.

Caffeine is a drug

Caffeine is a mild stimulant. It makes you feel more alert. It is found in coffee, and also in tea, cocoa, chocolate, and cola drinks. It's probably the world's most popular drug.

Caffeine is just like any other drug. The effect it has depends on your height, age, weight, and your body's own reaction to drugs. Caffeine may make you feel jittery and nervous. It can make you feel more awake, but you could have trouble sleeping too. Some people worry about the amount of caffeine they have every day. Because caffeine is a drug you may run into problems trying to give it up!

Amounts of caffeine in some drinks

Drink	Amount used	Caffeine in each small cup (140 ml)
Instant Coffee	rounded teaspoonful (1.5 g)	ranges from 54–72 mg
Decaffeinated Instant Coffee	rounded teaspoonful	about 5 mg
Ground coffee, percolated	rounded tablespoonful (7 g)	about 125 mg
Tea	rounded teaspoonful	50 mg
Cocoa	rounded teaspoonful	5 mg
Cola	small bottle (185 ml)	20 mg

Tobacco is a drug

How much do you know about smoking? There are 13 unlucky questions in the quiz below. This is because smoking is BAD NEWS.

1   The number of chemicals causing cancer in cigarettes is
(a) none   (b) 1
(c) 10   (d) 30

2   How many cigarettes do you need to smoke to raise your pulse rate?
(a) 1   (b) 5
(c) 10   (d) 25

3   Smoking is not permitted
(a) on underground trains
(b) in hospital wards
(c) in church
(d) in sports centres

4   Nicotine is a drug.
(a) true   (b) false

5   There is no point in stopping smoking because the damage is done.
(a) true   (b) false

6   A woman who smokes during her pregnancy can harm the baby.
(a) true   (b) false

7   Some people put on weight when they give up smoking.
(a) true   (b) false

8   Tobacco smoke can affect non-smokers as well as smokers.
(a) true   (b) false

9   This sign means
(a) don't smoke when driving
(d) ashtray
(c) do not smoke
(d) smokers only.

10   It is easy to tell a long-term smoker from a non-smoker. You can tell by their
(a) cough   (b) skin
(c) fingers   (d) teeth

11   Cigarette smoking is an addiction.
(a) true   (b) false

12   Smoking costs all tax-payers money.
(a) true   (b) false

13   Most young people who smoke will be killed by
(a) traffic accidents
(b) giving up smoking
(c) smoking cigarettes.

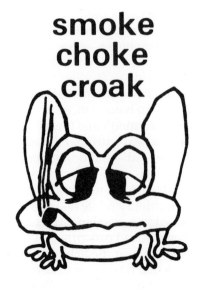

**smoke
choke
croak**

Answers

1 There are 30 known cancer-causing agents in cigarette smoke.
2 Just one, and straight after the first puff.
3 None of them allow smoking.
4 True. Nicotine is the drug in cigarettes. As you know, a drug is anything you put into your body which changes the way it works.
5 False. As soon as a smoker stops, the health risk decreases. The ex-smoker feels better, breathes easier, and can get fit again.
6 True. Babies born to mothers who smoke are likely to be underweight and not as strong as other babies.
7 True. Because their sense of smell improves and food tastes better.
8 True. Many non-smokers find that smoke irritates their eyes, nose, and throat. The smoke can be dangerous to those with chest or heart disease, or even be the cause of the disease.
9 Do not smoke. No words are given because this symbol is used all over the world. People know what it means no matter what their language.
10 All of them. Long-term smokers often have a chronic cough, stained fingers, wrinkly dull skin, and yellowish teeth.
11 True. Very few people can smoke only an occasional cigarette. Smoking is habit-forming and you can get addicted after only one or two weeks.
12 True. Hospitals are full of patients whose diseases are a direct result of smoking—heart disease, bronchitis, emphysema, and cancer of the mouth, throat, and lung. All taxpayers pay for hospital costs.
13 Cigarette smoking. Out of every 1000 male teenagers who smoke, one will later die violently, six will be killed on the roads, but 250 will be killed by smoking. No one gets killed by giving up smoking.

You can see that smoking really is BAD NEWS. And there's more! If you are a cigarette smoker you shorten your life by about 5½ *minutes* for each cigarette you smoke. How long does it take to smoke one? Why are cigarettes called 'coffin nails'?

Now the GOOD NEWS about smoking. The moment you stop smoking you start living longer and living better. And there is more good news! Your heart and lungs will work more efficiently and your blood will carry more oxygen. (You need all the oxygen your blood can carry for fitness.) You'll be less puffed and wheezy whenever you do something energetic and you won't get wrinkly and old-looking so soon.

You'll have more stamina, more staying power, food will taste better, you will get fewer colds and coughs and your resistance to illness will be better. You will be able to taste and smell better, and best of all you will feel fine.

Passive smoking

There are two types of smoke produced by a burning cigarette. One type, 'mainstream smoke', is filtered by the cigarette and inhaled by the smoker. The other type, 'sidestream smoke', goes directly into the air that others breathe. It is not filtered and so contains high concentrations of many of the substances which make cigarette smoking harmful. This makes it potentially dangerous to non-smokers.

Children are affected by sidestream smoke. Children in smoking households have decreased lung function and indications of small airways obstruction. They are more prone to serious chest illnesses like pneumonia and bronchitis and to general upper respiratory tract infections.

Passive smoking can also affect the child's future smoking behaviour. Research has shown that children are more likely to smoke if their parents do. Many children have their first cigarette at home. In one study 22% of children who smoked said that they first had a cigarette with their parents. Yet most parents report that they do not want their children to start smoking. They obviously do not realise that their own example has an important effect on their children's behaviour.

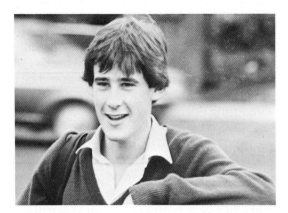

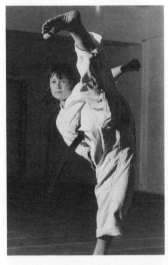

New Zealand Herald *photo*

'I began to notice that friends who smoked often had bad breath. They smelt of smoke and their clothes and hair did too. I didn't want to be like that.'

'I was aiming for a black belt and I was training hard. But I found I was getting out of breath. So I decided to give up smoking. I noticed the difference in just a few days. That was last year. Now I've got the black belt and I'm never going back to smoking.'

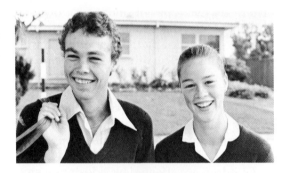

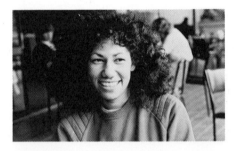

'Giving up smoking was the best thing we ever did. We decided to quit together and we helped each other. Now we have more fun, more money and we're not worrying about where the next smoke's coming from . . .'

'I'd never go out with anyone who smoked. I'd be scared if he smoked it would be like kissing an ash tray.'

These young people are all non-smokers.

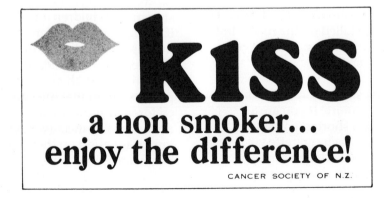

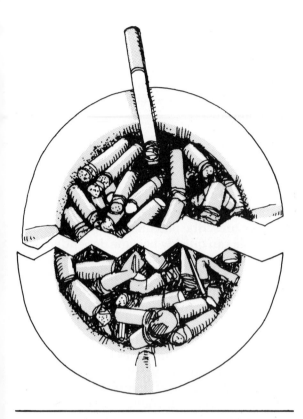

Breaking the cigarette habit means more fitness, cleaner breath (and therefore more sex appeal!) more money in the pocket, and less pollution in the air

produce interesting leaflets with plenty of handy hints to help you. Choose a good day to stop smoking, and get on with it! The sooner you stop the sooner you'll feel better about yourself.

Here are some more ways to hit the smoking habit.

- Plan to have lots to do.
- Learn some ways to relax.
- Do something active.
- Look in the mirror. Practise saying 'No thanks, I don't smoke.'
- Save the money you would have spent on cigarettes in a special place, ready to reward yourself for not smoking.
- Change your routines. Avoid situations where you'll be tempted to smoke.

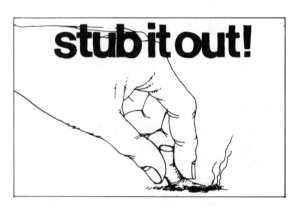

. . . an effective method to help you stop smoking!

Questions about giving up smoking

Q: Why do I find it hard to give up smoking?

Roger W.

A: Most smokers are *addicts*. But sometimes friends make them keep on smoking when they don't really want to.

Q: I've really had it. I want to be in charge of myself, not be ruled by that packet. Can you help me to give up smoking?

Jane

A: There's no one answer or method. Most experts think that giving up altogether is the only really successful way, rather than tapering off. The Health Education Council

Illegal drugs

Why do some people take drugs? We don't know exactly why. It could be for any of these reasons.

To rebel against parents and teachers.
Out of curiosity.
Because their friends pressured them.
To be like someone else.
To escape loneliness and boredom.
To relax.
To seem more sociable.
To escape family problems.

To avoid making decisions.
To stay alert or keep awake.
To identify with pop stars.
To be accepted in their circle of friends.
To overcome discomfort.
To escape from reality.
To get kicks.
To maintain a dependence.

People take drugs to alter their feelings, but there may be other effects as well. Every drug works on the body and mind in different ways to produce different effects. It helps to know what some of these effects can be.

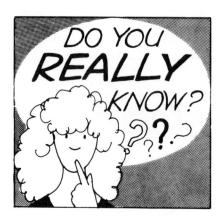

Hallucinogens

Hallucinogens affect a person's perceptions, awareness, and emotions. They are not usually addictive. L.S.D. is a very powerful hallucinogen. A person who uses L.S.D. can have a pleasant experience one time and a 'bad trip' or 'freak out' (a frightening experience) the next time he/she uses it. Some people who have used this drug have become mentally ill.

Marijuana is a mild hallucinogen thought to affect memory, sense of time, and performance.

Inhalants

Inhalants are a group of volatile substances, often household products, that are inhaled because of the effects that they produce. Use of them can cause ulcers of the nose and mouth, liver and kidney damage, blood disorders, permanent brain damage, or death. Frequently they are associated with confusion, slurred speech, headache, nausea, and vomiting.

Narcotics

Narcotics are drugs based on the opium poppy plant, and usually used as painkillers. Doctors prescribe narcotics with extreme care, as people can quickly become dependent on them. Narcotics include opium, morphine, heroin and codeine. Their effects vary from warm, floating feelings to nausea and lethargy. Experimenting with narcotics is likely to cause addiction. The cure for a person who becomes 'hooked' on a narcotic is very difficult and sometimes impossible, because withdrawal symptoms include mental effects, nausea, vomiting, diarrhoea, chilliness, sweating, cramps, and pain in the back and legs.

Sedatives

Small doses of sedatives are used to relax the user; larger doses will produce sleep. They are sometimes called 'downers'. A person can become addicted to sedatives. Barbiturates and tranquillisers are sedatives. So are sleeping pills.

A DEADLY COMBINATION:

Alcohol plus sedative equals:
- slowed-down breathing
- oxygen-starved brain
- permanent physical damage
- coma
- even death.

Stimulants

Stimulants speed up the body's actions. They are sometimes called 'uppers'. Cocaine is a strong stimulant. Amphetamines ('speed') are another. Use of these is risky; the user becomes anxious and unpredictable. They are addictive. Users develop sores and ulcers, infections, liver damage, and sometimes bleeding into the brain. 'Speed kills.'

We only know some of the effects of different drugs. But we do know that saying 'No' to drugs can make you feel good.

Saying 'No'

Turning down the chance to take or use a drug (alcohol, tobacco, marijuana, or anything else) is your RIGHT. Any friends who lean on you about your decision are trying to take away one of your rights as a free individual. You can remind them of that if they hassle you.

ACTIVITIES

1   There was a young lady from Gore
Who thought, 'To get better, take *more*.'
She drank all her potion,
some pills and cough lotion,
And now she's much worse than before.
If a little is good for you, is more better still?

2   (a) The sensible medicine code tells you to get rid of old pills or medicines by flushing them down the toilet or returning them to the chemist. What is wrong with throwing them in the rubbish tin?
(b) What are childproof bottles? Find out from a chemist what kinds are available.
(c) Find a prescription label and write the details in your exercise book. Does it have any special warnings on it?

3   Look in magazines for advertisements for herbal medicines. You could also look on the shelves in 'health food' shops and some supermarkets. List the names and the claims. Are any breaking the law?

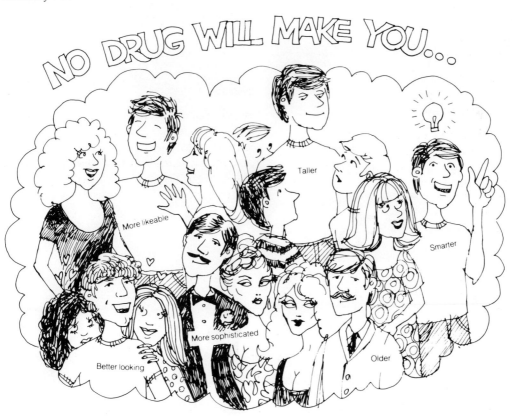

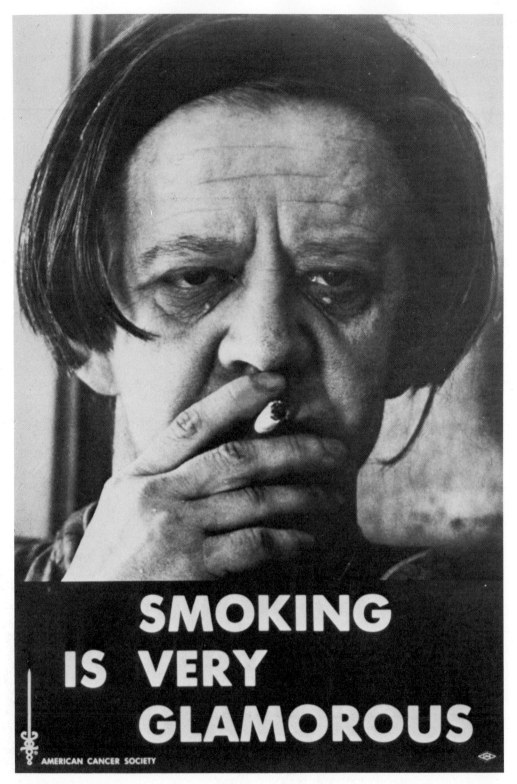

SMOKING IS VERY GLAMOROUS

AMERICAN CANCER SOCIETY

Reproduced with the permission of the American Cancer Society

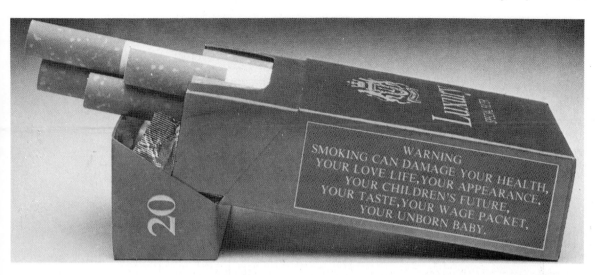

Courtesy of the Cancer Society of N.Z.

Caffeine

4 C - - - 'adds life' (Cola drink).
- - - - - - - - - - - - 'puts the life in you' (instant coffee)
Can these caffeine-containing drinks do this? Write jingles to advertise a caffeine-free soft drink or hot drink.

Smoking

5 What do you think are the most effective ways of discouraging people from starting to smoke?

6 Is smoking glamorous? Advertisers try to make cigarettes seem glamorous. They try to tell you that you will
 have more fun
 be more exciting (or manly or appealing)
 do better at sport
 be more successful
 look sophisticated
and have a clean taste in your mouth!
 Many of the tobacco companies aim their ads at young people, and women. Find and display advertisements for cigarettes. Decide what the advertiser is saying. What hidden messages can you find? What is the advertiser saying will happen to the smoker who smokes each brand?

7 Tobacco companies often sponsor sporting events. They are wealthy companies who can afford to give the sport the money it needs to survive. But smoking stops people from doing their best, because it affects their performance. Discuss or debate this strange situation.

8 How much does smoking cost? Find the price of a packet of cigarettes. Calculate how much a person smoking one packet a day pays. Now work out the cost per year. What could you buy with all this money?
 Find the warning on a real packet of cigarettes. Now compare it with the warning in the picture which is the front cover of a booklet put out by the Cancer Society. Which warning tells it like it really is? Why?

9 *Activity for smokers*
- Give up smoking for at least three days. Then pick out which of your friends and the people you meet are smokers (you will tell by the smell).
- Put the money you saved from not smoking into a jar. Buy yourself a reward (*not* cigarettes!).

10 What would *you* do? In small groups discuss:
- You have a sore throat. A friend has some pills the doctor prescribed for her. She offers you some
- At a party you're offered a cigarette. You haven't ever smoked before and are not sure if you know how
- You see someone put a pill in someone else's drink at the dance
- At the barbecue some of your group are passing a 'joint' (marijuana) around. It's passed to you.

11. In the United States codeine-containing pain relievers are not available. Why?

9
This side up, with care

You have nearly all the pieces you need to complete your health jigsaw. You are already making some good choices for yourself and your health. You are already feeling better for making those choices. But one piece of the jigsaw is missing.

You know your health needs (the things you can't live without). They are food, exercise, and cleanliness. But you can have the best food, the best exercise programme, and the cleanest body and still be miserable about yourself, because of that one missing piece.

This missing piece is about your mind, your feelings, and your emotions. People often say that it is wrong to be too concerned with yourself. They say things like

'young people are so selfish'

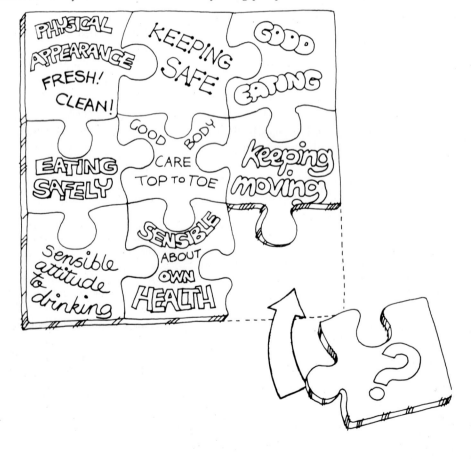

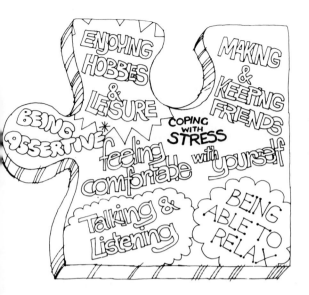

The missing piece . . .

'he doesn't care about anyone else'
'too much about self-knowledge in the education system today'.
But you must be concerned with yourself. You must know and like yourself! Until you can do this you will find it hard to be at ease with yourself and get on with other people.

You are important. But remember everyone else is the same. Each person is the most important person in the world.

> I'm important—you're important.

You have to remember this with everyone! Each one of your friends wants to be treated as important—boys and girls. Each person in your family wants to be treated as important. So does everyone else you meet.

You don't like it when others put you down and make you feel:
inferior
less than OK
stupid
clumsy
or dumb.

No one else likes it either. Sometimes *you* are the one who puts you down. It's important to keep this in mind:

> I am a worthwhile person.

There are some things about you which you don't like. But that doesn't mean you are a rotten person.

Sometimes you will feel happy and comfortable with yourself. Other times you may feel unhappy. Your feelings about yourself and your relationships will be better if you can let other people know how you feel and can understand their feelings too. You have to practise this. Your family and friends aren't in the guessing game! Hints or clues are not enough:

- Wayne said he didn't want to go to school because he felt sick, but really he was trying to tell his Dad that he was having problems at school.

- Lindy would never take any of her friends home. She pretended her mother had said she wasn't allowed. But really Lindy was terrified her mother would be drunk in front of her friends.

- Amy told Dillon that she wasn't allowed to go out with him. But really she was scared of going out with him.

Let's try these again . . .

- Wayne felt miserable about school. He wanted help and support, and to talk over his problem with somebody. In the end he waited till his Dad relaxed and then he said, 'Dad, I need your help. Please listen to me. I want to tell you how I feel.'

- Lindy felt ashamed of her mother. Lindy went to Alateen and discovered that she was really ashamed of her mother's *sickness*. Lindy learnt ways of coping, and now she says: 'My mother is ill. She has a disease which she has to face up to'. . . Lindy's friends like Lindy for herself.

---

* To be assertive means recognising your own abilities and letting others know your feelings and needs. It does not mean being aggressive, angry, or selfish.

• Amy *was* scared of going out with Dillon. She said to him, 'I don't like the way you drive. It makes me feel frightened.' Dillon got the message.

. . . Wayne, Lindy, and Amy have learnt how to be assertive. They don't expect family members or friends to guess their feelings any longer.

Body language

Sometimes people can tell how you are feeling by how you look and act. This is called body language. You can let your feelings be known without speaking.

You are reading body language all the time. Try reading the language in the pictures below and opposite. Alongside each picture is a set of statements. Decide which best describes the feelings involved.

Even though you are always reading body language, sometimes it's hard to be quite sure what the message is. You might:

Shrug your shoulders (don't know? don't care?)

Wink at someone (funny joke? hello? see you later?)

Yawn openly (boring? tired? stuffy?)

Turn away (shy? fed up? closing the discussion?)

Pat someone on the back (well done? friendly? condescending?)

1 Anne-Marie is
    upset
    happy
    bored
    lonely
    daydreaming
    tired.

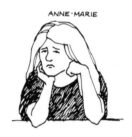
ANNE-MARIE

2 Gill is
    unhappy
    puzzled
    pregnant
    sleepy
    daydreaming.

Les is
    not interested
    concerned
    angry.

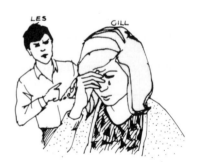
LES   GILL

3 Dad is
    listening willingly
    going to say no
    approving.

Mum is
    puzzled
    calming Dad
    not interested.

Gray is
    calm
    demanding something
    happy.

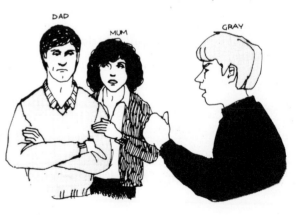
DAD   MUM   GRAY

4 Pete
    is part of the Group
    is lonely
    hates the Group
    wishes he belonged to the Group.

  The Group
    are friends
    are talking about Pete.

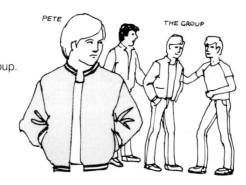

All these people are showing how they feel with body language

Friends

Some people find it quite easy to make friends, but most of us need to make an effort. You may have said to yourself that you must 'join something and meet more people'. It's easy to think that people won't like you or that you haven't got much to offer. But every single person is a worthwhile person who is unique. Everyone has lots of strengths, talents, and abilities and is in some way interesting. The thing is to find those qualities in yourself and others. If you find this hard, try listing your own good points.

Some classes have tried this sort of exercise: each person makes up a self-advertisement highlighting his or her
    unique features
    special qualities
    physical characteristics
    special abilities
    things they've achieved.
Lawrence's ad is shown on page 96.
Once you know that you have something worthwhile to offer, make an effort and get to know some new people. Try some of these tips:

- Always look a person in the eye as you talk. This is called **eye contact**
- Introduce yourself to a new person at school, where you work, or at the local shops. Just say, 'Hello, I'm (Paul/Paula).

You're new aren't you?' or 'Have you been here long?' Show interest in what the person says to you

- Ask someone if you can borrow something. Arrange to return it, and return it on time
- Start a conversation with the person next to you when you're next waiting for service somewhere
- Offer to help someone
- Hold a small party for 3–5 people. Invite at least one person you don't know, or ask a friend to invite someone new
- Say 'hello' today to three people you meet—ones you wouldn't usually speak to. Try to get a smile and a return 'Hello' from them.

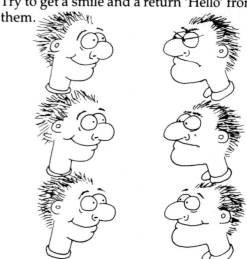

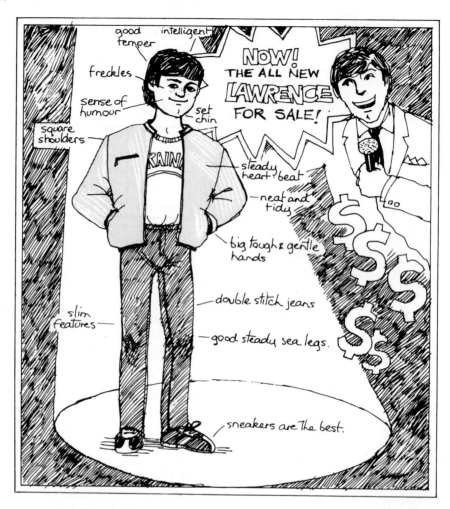

How can you show people that you are their friend?

At home, try this.

1   Imagine you are not allowed to do something you really want to. Let your face show how you feel. Now let your mirror see that face.

2   Think of the very best thing that ever happened to you. Let your face remember how good you felt.

Look in the mirror again. Which is the face you like best? Which face would you rather see at breakfast time? In the street?

Now you can show people that you are their friend.

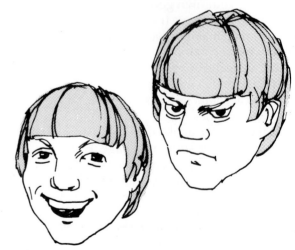

● Remember the smiling face you saw in the mirror? People appreciate a warm and friendly smile.

- Try to think of something kind to say.
- Make a phone call to let your friends know you are interested in them.
- Show your friends you are thinking of them. Write a note or a letter, just to show you care.
- Make or do something for a friend.

The support and friendship of other people is vital to you to keep you the 'right side up', so that your mental and emotional needs are met. In the same way your support and friendship is vital to those other people.

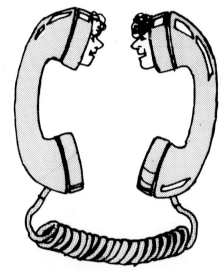

Telephone a friend today!

Stress

Things don't always go right. People have to expect some upsets or difficulties in their lives. These upsets make demands on your body. Your body responds to demands made on it—whether pleasant or unpleasant—in these ways:

　　your heart beats quickly
　　your stomach 'lurches'
　　your face flushes
　　you sweat
　　you are tense.

The tiny adrenal glands behind the kidneys send energy-activating adrenalin pouring into your system. Your muscles prepare for action. . . fight? or flight? In ancient times when people were faced with dangers like cave bears, the fight or flight reaction was useful. They could either run away fast, or stand and fight. When the danger passed, their bodies returned to normal.

Nowadays people don't usually have to fight bears for a home! But their bodies still have to cope with stressful situations:

　　waiting for an exciting event
　　lining up for a race
　　a near car-crash
　　watching a suspenseful movie
　　an argument with a close friend
　　an illness, accident, or death.

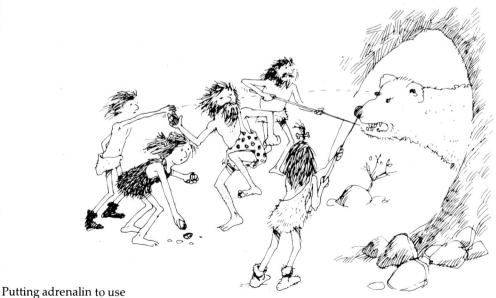

Putting adrenalin to use

Stress is normal. In fact your life would be dull and boring if you had no stress at all. Stress only becomes a problem if you have too much, too often.

Nowadays we can't remove our stress by running away, or fighting. We have to do something else, because too much stress can damage the body. Some signs can warn that your body is under too much stress. You:

Feel tired all the time, even when you seem to be getting enough sleep

Keep getting colds and other minor illnesses

Get vague aches and pains which have no real cause

Over-react (get very angry for little reason)

Might stop caring about things altogether or get over-anxious

May eat, drink, or smoke too much.

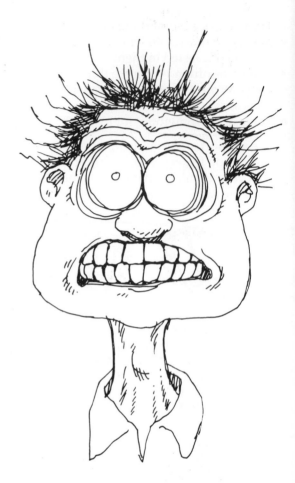

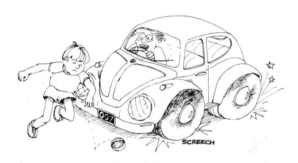

In modern life we can feel stress, but have no way to 'work it off'.

What can you do about too much stress?

If you're feeling stressful, you could

bite your nails
light a cigarette
snap at somebody
cry
take a tranquilliser
have a drink
shout
eat something
chew a pencil
hit somebody.

You *could*, but it won't help you to cope with stress. *You must do something positive about your stress.*

Here are some ways of coping with stress.

- *Breathe deeply.* Sit or lie quietly for at least five minutes. Breathe in, then hold your breath for a moment, then breathe out slowly. (Some yoga breaths are like this.)
- *Talk to yourself.* Sit or lie down. Talk to yourself. Say words like calm, peaceful, quiet, still, relax, rest, comfortable, gentle. . . .
- *Walk.* Just a walk will help use up the extra energy the adrenalin released. Try just walking away for a few minutes, whenever you feel stressed.
- *Tense up/relax.* Tense up different parts of your body one after the other, then relax them.

tense toes . . . relax
tense feet . . . relax
tense calves . . . relax
and so on until you are relaxed all over.

- *Listen to music.* Choose relaxing music!
- *Do something energetic.* Dig the garden—take the dog out—go for a jog.
- *Meditate.* Repeat a syllable like 'OM' to yourself as you sit with eyes closed.
- *Find a regular exercise programme or hobby*
Here are some ideas:
Granny used to sweep the stairs if she was upset
Peter does a work-out at the gym every lunch time
Doug swims two kilometres every morning
Lynne 'goes flop' on her bed for a few minutes
Dave chops wood if he's cross
Jacquie uses yoga to relax her before exams
Ed has a warm bath and plays the transistor to calm himself down

Jill does TM (Transcendental Meditation)
Ken works on his model trains
Lorna always has half an hour alone every day—she sits or lies quietly.

You can make changes in your lifestyle to reduce stress.

Do one thing at a time. Sort out what has to be done, and how you will do it. Leave things that don't matter.

Be thoughtful and friendly. This will make other people respond to you and make a happier, more relaxed environment.

Don't bottle things up. Talk your problems over with someone you trust.

Learn to relax. Make time to relax every day.

Make time to enjoy something you like every day. Work on your hobby—have some time to yourself.

Take a break! When things aren't going well, stop and do something else.

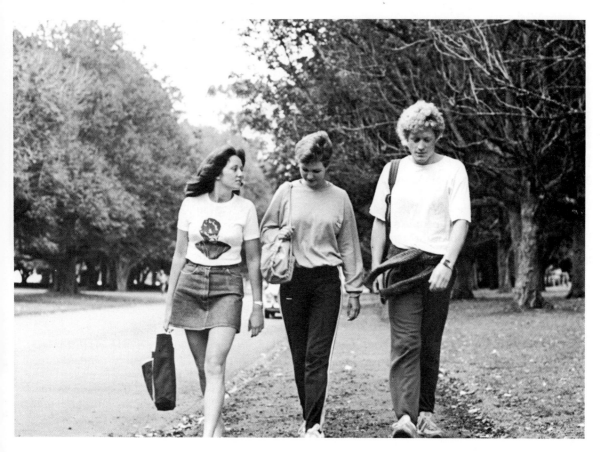

Get enough sleep. No one can cope with stress if they're short of sleep.

Exercise regularly. Exercise makes you feel good. Some experts think that exercise releases special chemicals called endorphins which give you a natural 'high'.

Care for yourself. You are the only person who can really care for your own self. Of course you need other people, but you are the one who is in charge of your

　　choices
　　decisions
　　and actions.

To feel fine, make the decisions you know will be best for you.

You are going to change. In weeks or months you will notice some differences. All your friends will be changing, too. New things will happen.

ACTIVITIES

1　Arrange for someone to come to talk to the class about Assertiveness Training. You may be able to arrange a whole course for those who are interested.

2　Mime different feelings to the class. Get your 'body language' message across. No speaking allowed by the actors! Try such feelings as angry, bored, miserable, fed up, pleased, and afraid.

3　'Assertive people let others know their feelings.'
　　'Sometimes you have to tell little lies.'
　　'It's wrong to hurt other people's feelings.'
Can all these statements be right? Discuss.

4　Discuss these statements.
'The person who loses his temper is always the loser.'
'You're like an open book.'
'Actions speak louder than words.'

5　What is a friend? Finish these statements.
'I think a friend is . . . .'
'I think a friend should not . . . .'

6　The way we see ourselves is known as our **self image**. We try to look at the good things about ourselves and build up a positive self image. Write down

- Something you like about an ancestor of yours
- Something you like about what you were like or did when you were little
- Something you like about where you are living or your surroundings
- Something you like about your talents, ability, or what you inherited
- Something you like about your body or what it can do
- Something you like about you, your personality, or emotions
- You are good at . . . .

The way we see ourselves affects how other people see us.

7　In your exercise book use a whole page to do a self-advertisement for a magazine or newspaper. Be sure to highlight all the best, positive, good, caring, different, and interesting things about you and what you have done. Include any certificates, awards, exams.

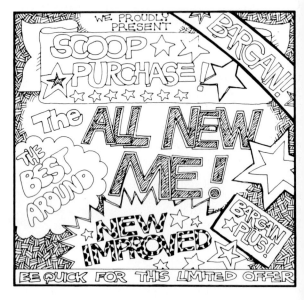

8　(a)　How is yoga breathing done? What else does yoga offer?
(b)　What does TM (Transcendental Meditation) involve?

9　A Stress chart has been developed by some American doctors to test stress levels in adults. People score 0 for all 'no' answers, and add up all their 'yes' points. If a person scores under 150 he or she is not over-stressed. If the person scores between 150–300 points they are quite stressed. Over 300 points? The person is at risk from stress-related illness.

Life event	Answer		Point value
Death of spouse	yes	no	100
Divorce	yes	no	73
Jail term	yes	no	63
Death of close family member	yes	no	63
Personal injury or illness	yes	no	53
Marriage	yes	no	50
Fired from work	yes	no	47
Marital reconciliation	yes	no	45
Retirement	yes	no	45
Pregnancy	yes	no	40
Change in financial status	yes	no	38
Change of work	yes	no	36
Mortgage or loan over $20,000	yes	no	31
Trouble with in-laws	yes	no	29
Outstanding personal achievement	yes	no	28
Trouble with boss	yes	no	23
Change in residence	yes	no	20
Change in social activities	yes	no	18
Change in number of family gatherings	yes	no	15
Vacation	yes	no	13
Christmas season	yes	no	12
Minor violation of the law	yes	no	11

Which things would be most stressful to you and other teenagers? Make up a chart. There is no need to give points.

11   Look up a copy of the contract you made at the beginning of this book. How have you got on since? Will you need to make a new contract? Write it down in your book.

Index